595HD

DRUG
DEPENDENCE

DRUG
DEPENDENCE
aspects of ego function

Henry Krystal, M.D.
Herbert A. Raskin, M.D.
WAYNE STATE UNIVERSITY

Wayne State University Press   Detroit   1970

*Published simultaneously in Canada by
The Copp Clark Publishing Company
517 Wellington Street, West
Toronto 2B, Canada.*

*LC catalog card 76–121920
ISBN 0–8143–1419–8*

contents

Preface	7
Introduction	9
I Affect Tolerance	15
A Genetic View of Affects	15
Pain and anxiety	16
Theory of the developmental history of affects	20
Affect disturbance in drug dependence	22
The Problem of Trauma	29
The stimulus barrier	31
Stimulus barrier and affect tolerance	32
Use of drugs in augmenting stimulus barrier	33
Case illustration	35
Effect of trauma on affect tolerance	36
Drugs and the Pleasure-Pain Principle	38
Thrills and regressions of affect	38
The principle of constancy	39
"Corruption" of life enhancing functions of the erotogenic zones	41
The relief principle	43
II Object-Representation and Self-Representation	45
Placebo Studies	45
The Object and Object-Representation	47
Nature of the repressed object	49

Object-Representation and Self-Representation in
    Depression   52
    Object-representation in schizophrenia   55
Résumé of Object-Representation in Drug
    Dependence   58
    Case illustrations   58
Review of the Concept of Repression   64
The Handling of Aggression and its Effect on Self-
    Representation and Object-Representation   67
Summary   70

**III Dealing with Emotions by Modification of
Consciousness**   73
Altered States of Consciousness   75
Orientation versus Disorientation   79
Wakefulness to Sleep States Spectrum   85
Self-Awareness   87
    Modification of superego function   89
    Case illustration   92
    Modification of body image and body function   93
Summary   95

IV Implications for Therapy   97
A Preparatory Phase of Treatment Serving to
    Increase Affect Tolerance   99
The Prohibition by Command and Pharmacological
    Agents   102
The Problem of Counter-Transference   103
Facilitating the Establishment of a Benign Introject   104
Solo Therapy versus Treatment in a Clinic   107
Aggression in Drug Dependent Individuals   108

References   113
Index   120

preface

This monograph has been in preparation for several years. Observations have been culled from extensive psychotherapy and psychoanalysis with drug dependent individuals, even though few specific cases are reported. Dr Raskin's experience has involved directing the Detroit Narcotics Clinic from 1953 to 1967; Dr Krystal was director of the Highland Park Alcoholism Treatment Center from 1955 to 1962. During this time, an inspiration to our work was a seminar on depression conducted by Dr John M. Dorsey at the Department of Psychiatry of the Detroit Receiving Hospital (now Detroit General Hospital).

Chapter I is a revision of a paper entitled "Anxiety and Pain Tolerance," read to the December 1964 meeting of the American Psychoanalytic Association in New York, and in October 1964 to a meeting of the Detroit Psychoanalytic Society. Chapter II was modified after a paper read to the December 1965 meeting of the American Psychoanalytic Association in New York.

Special appreciation is expressed to Drs Thomas A. Petty, Max Warren, and Channing T. Lipson, who together with the authors constituted a study group in which these matters were discussed repeatedly. Dr John Dorsey offered his criticism and suggestions so generously that it is impossible to credit him with all the ideas derived from him.

We also wish to thank Dorothy Eckert and Rose Russ for their preparation of this work for publication.

H.K.
H.A.R.

Detroit, Michigan
September 1969

introduction

It was not many years ago that defining "addiction" was a relatively simple matter. It always meant "drug addiction," and this almost invariably meant opiate addiction, most usually heroin. It described a physical or physiological dependence upon the drug substance, a vague reference to some kind of psychological or emotional dependence, the factor of tolerance, and most important, the abstinence or withdrawal syndrome. Without strict adherence to these four criteria, "addiction" did not exist; the person would be "habituated" or "using."

Unfortunately, increasing knowledge of a subject frequently seems to confound and complicate it. We are all aware that our old term "addiction" has grown far beyond its mere allusion to the abuse of narcotic drug substances. The list of "addicting" depressant, stimulant and hallucinogenic drugs continues to grow each day. This is not to mention the idea of "addiction" to such things as food, cigarettes, coffee, people, sex and love. Even our old definition of drug addiction has fallen in terms of increased tolerance and physiological dependence.

The Expert Committee on Drugs Liable to Produce Addiction, World Health Organization, took the first step away from archaic thinking. In 1957 the World Health Organization adopted this revised definition:

Drug addiction is a state of periodic or chronic intoxication detrimental to the individual and to society, produced by the repeated consumption of a drug (natural or synthetic). Its characteristics include: (1) an overpowering desire or need (compulsion) to continue taking the drug and to obtain it by any means; (2) a *tendency* to increase the dose; (3) a psychic (psychological) and *sometimes* a physical dependence on the effects of the drug. (121) [*Italics ours*]

The psychological elements inherent in the particular relationship established between the person and his drug finally gained their proper focus. The physical dependence, abstinence, or withdrawal syndrome became a "sometimes" thing; tolerance became a "tendency" to increase the dose of the drug. These characteristics came to be viewed as only complications and elaborations of the nature and chemical structure of the particular drug involved and the dose and frequency with which it was used. Innumerable physical, physiological, and social conditions were observed to be consequences and outgrowths of the syndrome, often serving as strong reinforcements of the process but not the primary cause.

But, even this cannot be so simply stated. Krystal, in dealing with the withdrawal syndrome as a state of stress, has shown that the consideration of intrapsychic institutions and of multiple psychophysiological factors is indispensable to its proper understanding (61).

The more recent change in terminology from "drug addiction" to "drug dependence," as so eruditely recommended by Eddy *et al.* in 1965 (122), represents another major step toward a more accurate understanding of the "addictive process." It has finally come to be recognized that its etiology resides in the psychological structure and functioning of the human being, rather than in the pharmacological effect of the drug. We are dealing with sick people and the drug is not the problem but is an attempt at a self-help that fails.

At the present time the phenomenon of drug dependence cannot be completely explained or even understood. There is more that we do not know than we do know. A true understanding of drug dependence will not evolve until we can more adequately correlate psychodynamic and psychopathologic functioning of the human being as an individual organism and as a member of a group, psychosociological and physical environmental characteristics, and psychopharmacological and neurophysiological interrelationships.

The drug dependent person constitutes a particularly unique type of problem to himself and to society. Drug dependence is a medical syndrome, a chronic relapsing symptom complex invariably reflecting some form of underlying mental disturbance. The drug dependent person is suffering from a serious mental or emotional disorder and manifests this disorder in great part through his craving for and his relationship to the drug substance. The meaning of this reaching out for the drug, the dependence and reliance upon it, is seen to vary from patient to patient. The drug can be observed to serve different functions at different times even within the same person. Drug dependence is seen to be operative in patients attempting to deal with anxiety, guilt, aggression, inadequacy, depression, loneliness and longing, sexual urges, perversions, physical pain, psychoses, neuroses, and character disorders.

In the course of our work and research with drug dependence, it came to be held by some of us that drug dependence represented a manifestation of ego function, a mode of adaptation, perhaps the sole adjustive mechanism to living problems the person has available to himself at the moment. It constitutes that person's attempt to help himself, literally to live himself in the best way he can. It is held to be a symptom representation, a behavioristic reflection of some sort of psychological stress-functioning, an attempt to meet, deal with or master some form of intrapsychic imbalance, conflict or excitation. It is a kind of last-grasping toward something so as to forestall the horror of the feeling of inevitable disintegration of self, of psychic disorganization that spells the doom of total helplessness.

In their monumental studies of the adolescent "drug addict" in New York, Isidor Chein, Donald L. Gerard, Robert S. Lee, and Eva Rosenfeld place in clear perspective the manifold characteristics of the drug dependent person with two major propositions:

"(1) The addiction of the adolescent studied was an extension of, or a development out of, long-lasting, severe, personality disturbance and maladjustment. (2) The addiction of the adolescents we have studied was adaptive, functional, and dynamic." These studies also demonstrate the validity that "the probability of addiction is greater if the person experiences changes in his situation in connection with his use of opiate drugs which may be described as adaptive, functional, or ego syntonic and which he describes in terms which tell us that he regards the use of opiates as extremely worth while despite, or perhaps especially because of, the inconveniences and difficulties of being an addict in our society" (17).

The concepts of ego psychology have been presented in many well-known psychoanalytic studies. These have dealt with the almost limitless number and types of ego functions, both as related to intrapsychic conflict genesis and the conflict-free ego sphere. It is obviously beyond our intent here to review the wealth of these studies and how all ego functions relate directly to the phenomenon of drug dependence. It has been our experience, however, in meeting with patients from both clinic and private practice, to observe certain areas of ego functioning that seemed to us to be especially pertinent to the pathogenesis and continuing clinical existence of such a state. We have become particularly impressed with three such areas: (1) the ego vis-à-vis affects, especially anxiety and depression, (2) object-representation and self-representation, and (3) modifications of consciousness. Reflections on theoretical clinical observations of these areas of ego function and ego dysfunction in the drug dependent person constitute the essential theme of this report.

I

affect tolerance

There are few generalizations which can be stated to be applicable to drug dependence. A striking exception is that the drug dependent person invariably is seeking relief, modification or avoidance of a painful state. In his drug he has found something that he knows will put an end to unbearable tensions, pain. His own ego resources, organization, and functions suffer from impairments and defects which produce an insidious and inexorable helplessness to deal with pain and tension without his drug. But pain and painful affects are very complex phenomena. Preliminary to our study of painful affects will be a review of some work on pain.

A GENETIC VIEW OF AFFECTS

It is generally assumed that the degree of physical pain experienced is proportional to the extent of the injury. Such is not the case, however, even in those body areas adequately supplied with pain fibers. Physiological and psychological studies made since World War II have shown that the experience of pain is inseparable from anxiety, pain anticipation anxiety and fear of destruction of one's self (114). The relation of anxiety to problems of aggression, object-representations (benign introject), and the development of the ability to desomatize and verbalize affect, seems to be closely related to the development of drug dependence.

It is the anxiety associated with pain that provides its unbearable quality (72 79). It is the anxiety mobilized which threatens to overwhelm all other perceptions and functions of the entire self, but especially to overwhelm conscious ego functions. Anxiety and pain are very closely related. Each state is modified and influenced by the other. Exposure to much pain is likely to produce excessive anxiety, and the presence of anxiety almost invariably predisposes to and increases pain response.

Pertinent here is Melzack's observation that before a surgical procedure people will rarely ask, "how deeply, how extensively will you cut me?" but rather, "how much will it hurt?" (79). Here anxiety is motivated by the fear of pain, rather than of the injury for which the pain stands. The close and persistent connection between pain and anxiety can also be illustrated by a unique disturbance in individuals with congenital pain agnosia, in their ability to anticipate danger.

A review of the literature on the subject indicates that many such individuals keep hurting themselves accidentally, or perform in side-shows and have various sharp articles driven into their flesh. Their psychic reality is devoid of fear and pain and they generally show a lack of normal anxiety reactions or empathy with other people's anxiety. An interesting example is that of a famous performer who regularly had nails and pins driven into his tongue and other parts of his body. He arranged for "a spectacular," his own crucifixion. After a couple of gold-plated nails had been hammered into his hands and feet, the show had to be discontinued because of the massive incidence of fainting in the audience. The performer was totally surprised (21).

In "congenital analgesic indifference" there is a hyporeactivity to pain, apparently an underestimation of danger and subsequently inadequate utilization and function of anxiety as a signal. The opposite is ordinarily true of severely traumatized individuals. They often show intensity as a permanent character trait plus chronic anxiety states (116). Additionally, studies on concentration camp survivors found that many of them hyperreact to pain in a practically hypochondriacal fashion. Pain mobilizes dream-screens of their trauma. If they develop pain while asleep, they dream of the return of the trauma (e.g., of being in a concentration camp in a situation of great peril). This is the result of the formation of a type of screen memory, the traumatic screen (64). Once a traumatic screen is established, pain mobilizes all the anxiety of impending traumatization, and as the dreams of the concentration camp survivors show, pain is experienced as the return of the traumatic situation. We can also add that in *massive* psychic traumatization a reaction is established similar to that described by Greenacre regarding traumatization in infancy and the prenatal period (44). The result is that pain and/or danger mobilize excessive amounts of anxiety, especially its somatic component (64).

In normal people the introduction of small amounts of anxiety (e.g., preoperatively) raises the threshold of trauma resistance. There has been extensive experimentation in desensitizing soldiers to fears provoked by front-line explosions and by dangers in war-games (102). But in both of these situations, an excess of anxiety, noise or pain will panic and demoralize the patient or trainee, rendering him later incapable of tolerating even small quantities of pain or anxiety.

Physicians especially tend to think of the problem of pain in terms of the pain threshold, with the idea that neurotic, anxious patients perceive pain where others do not. Besides the fact that it is simpler to measure pain threshold, the attitude reflects the doctor's experience and belief that only the patients who complain of pain have it. The fact is that the problem is that of the ability to *tolerate* pain, and it is in this sphere that the amount of anxiety accompanying the pain is the essential factor. This applies to physical pain, "mental pain," which indicates the pain experience not generated in a diseased organ, and painful affects (96). Perhaps only in a lobotomized patient (or one chemically lobotomized) is the experience of pain not associated with anxiety, and therefore does not become unbearable.

From studies in the use of narcotic analgesics it is now quite evident that they do not provide relief from pain but from the attending anxiety. In experimental subjects, if pain is experienced without the feeling of danger (anxiety), no relief is obtained from narcotics (10). In clinical patients the relief of pain with narcotics is abolished by the injection of sympatho-mimetic drugs (119). Morphine was shown to reduce the disruptive effect of pain upon performance which was associated with anxiety produced by the anticipation of pain (50). The studies of Goldstein indicate that even aspirin has an anxiety relieving effect, "similar to those of minor tranquilizing drugs and small doses of phenobarbital" (43).

What then, is the genesis of this close relationship between pain and anxiety; what are its genetic antecedents? Anna Freud commented:

> Where the direct observation of infants in the first year of life is concerned, the relative proportion of physiological and psychological elements in the experience of pain is an open question. At this stage, any tension, need or frustration is probably felt as "pain," no real distinction being made yet between the diffuse experience of discomfort and the sharper and more circumscribed one of real pain arising from specific sources. In the first months of life, the threshold of resistance against stimulation is low and painful sensations assume quickly the dignity of traumatic events. (34)

Traumatization at this early stage, before physical pain is recognized and identified as a specific kind of disturbance, also poses some questions regarding the effect of trauma prior to the development of adequate reflective self-awareness. The point is the trauma may interfere with the very development of a fine discrimination between what is truly dangerous and what is not, what is external and what is internal. Khan has pointed out that the mother supplements the infant's stimulus barrier in her protective function. When pain develops, the child's security is threatened with a failure of the magical protection from the omnipotent love object (55). The reactions here are complex, and include aggression and guilt. Pain thereafter retains the ability to mobilize the threat of failure of the remnants and transferences of the maternal protection.

Theory of the developmental history of affects

Krystal's studies of drug withdrawal states led him to suggest that anxiety and depression evolve from a common precursor (Ur-affect) (61). In a drug dependent person there is a regression in regard to affects, anxiety and depression are again de-differentiated and show other attributes of primitivisation of affects, such as resomatization, deverbalization. The ideational component of the affect is isolated from its expressive aspects (glandular and muscular responses). The affects are experienced as threatening and therefore excluded from conscious awareness whenever possible. All of these characteristics, especially the regression to the "all or none" affective responses, impair their use as signals. We will presently attempt to discuss these in detail.

Prior to the "discovery" of the love object, the infant's response to distress takes a single form: totally somatic and uncontrollable. The establishment of the nuclei of self-representation and object-representation facilitates the separation of pain from the painful affects, which remain as a single, totally somatic reaction to the absence and threat of loss of the love object. In addition, the infant's physiological balance is so precarious, and lability so great, that affective disturbance produces immediate physical changes and pain. Anxiety in the infant may produce instant colic and hence be converted into severe pain. Other affects can similarly be converted into painful physical symptoms, because the infant lacks the adult's protective ego functions and is more readily thrown into psychogenic shock which may be lethal. This type of reaction accounts for the child's confrontation with mortal fear; not fear of dying, but an enormous, overwhelming, deadly anxiety of being eaten up, swallowed, etc. This death anxiety is linked with the feeling of helplessness, immobility, suffocation, and remains the core of that overwhelming anxiety which in the adult we refer to as the "automatic anxiety" in trauma: castration anxiety, fear of dismemberment, losing one's mind (28). Perhaps it is also what Melanie Klein called "psychotic anxiety" linked with the ideational component of the fear of falling to bits. This feeling is unbearable, and is the thing that causes, or more properly, is the traumatic situation. It initiates a series of unconscious pathogenic reactions which represent the trauma syndrome.

Out of the infant's general state of distress, several states and feelings evolve. The "discovery" of the mother and her power to nurture and give relief shifts the ideational component of it from physical distress to the fear of the loss of the object. This shift establishes the basis for the object-representation in the child's mind which we will discuss in detail in Chapter II.

With the increased acuity of perception and the maturation of the ego apparatuses of proprioception, the body image is gradually built up. Pain is separated from the general distress pattern, albeit it is never completely separated from anxiety. Still, the normal adult does not obtain automatic relief from physical pain by oral gratification. Some of this potential, however, is retained, as we shall demonstrate in our discussion of the placebo. This type of reaction is one of the remnants of infantile function which becomes important in drug dependence.

As to other affects, anxiety becomes separated from depression primarily in the fact that anxiety is the reaction to the expectation of danger, whereas depression represents a hopeless giving up and resignation. The "agitation" in anxiety serves an expressive function, and when the situation is hopeless, a flaccid or tense-immobile catatonoid, inhibited reaction develops (105). Depression and anxiety not only become separated but also become in a way antagonistic because of their physiologic association with opposing parts of the autonomic nervous system. Thus, it happens that sometimes either on order of physicians or in drug self-medication, people can stimulate the anxiety-agitation response (with amphetamine drugs or fear-producing thrills) as a way to combat the parasympathetic aspects of depression.

Affect disturbance in drug dependence

However, in many drug dependent persons we find an affect combining depression and anxiety, a disturbance in which the de-differentiation of anxiety and depression takes place or a state in which the differentiation was never successfully accomplished. Thus, in Krystal's studies of drug withdrawal states, the affect seemed to approximate the infantile "total" and somatic distress pattern rather than a clear-cut adult affect pattern (61). Rado was the first to describe this condition clinically, calling it "the anxious depression" of alcoholics (95). He did not, however, pursue in detail the nature and consequences of this regression. Engel considers "anxiety and depression withdrawal" to be the "primary affect of unpleasure" (28). His excellent and scholarly work traces the development of the Ur-affects in the infant in relation to drives and object representations, and confirms the expressive attitudes of anxiety ("flight or fight") and depression ("to give up") to be a psychological continuum, although they "represent two basic physiological states." He pointed out that depressions may become "maladaptive or unsuccessful in which case they seem to be potent provoking conditions for major psychic and somatic disorganizations, sometimes leading to death."

Perhaps Freud also hinted at this developmental history of the painful affects when he said about the infant's reaction to loss, in the "Problems of Anxiety," that "some things were fused together which later will be separated. He is not yet able to distinguish temporary absence from permanent loss" (38). Shur has come to similar conclusions about the development of affects and has drawn our attention to the fact that affects like other aspects of mental function, are subject to regression. Schur's work on the metapsychology of fear contributed the observation of a type of *physiological regression* in patients with dermatoses, which allows us to add another dimension to our knowledge of some drug dependent individuals. We gain an appreciation of a regression manifest in the words of Schur in "a regressive evaluation of danger and an ego which responds with deneutralized energy. This corresponds to the re-emerging somatic discharge phenomena." Upon observing that some patients developed symptoms representing anxiety equivalents instead of becoming conscious of their anxiety, Schur postulated that there was an "interdependence" between the ego's faculty to use secondary processes and neutralized energy, and the desomatization response (105). This implies an inverse relation between an individual's consciousness of his affect and the intensity of physiological (stress) responses and affect equivalents. The relevance of the *regression* vis-à-vis the problem of pain consists in the nature of pain, which is a complex conscious phenomenon composed of the perception of injury associated with disturbing affects. Commonly the affect involved is that of anxiety. However, in the regressed state the impact of the resomatized Ur-affect presents a complex danger. One of the results, which will be discussed in detail later, is the inability to tolerate even small amounts of anxiety, hence the failure of its signal function. This creates the threat of trauma, to which we shall return.

A reconsideration of the mode of development of the affect of anxiety from the infantile, that is, totally somatic, to the adult form suggests that the original pattern is modified by later experiences and developments. Verbalization and desomatization of affect represent one aspect of ego development (105). Learned responses to pain as the representative of danger represent another and important aspect. We will pursue the story of development of pain tolerance in the child, because it can serve us as a pattern and prototype for the development of individual resources for dealing with painful states and affects.

Pain is a perceptive process in which the possibility of injury is evaluated in terms of one's psychic reality. Anna Freud, in considering the effect of pain on children, observed:

> According to the child's interpretation of the event, young children react to pain not only with anxiety but with other affects appropriate to the contents of the unconscious phantasies, i.e., on the one hand with anger, rage and revenge feelings, on the other with masochistic submission, guilt or depression . . . and . . . where anxiety derived from phantasy plays a minor or no part, even severe pain is borne well and forgotten quickly. Pain augmented by anxiety, on the other hand, even if slight in itself, represents a major event in the

child's life and is remembered long afterward, the memory being frequently accompanied by phobic defenses against its possible return. (34)

Here, Anna Freud treats pain as an absolute perception, indicating that the child's responses to it are modified by the factors stated. We would maintain, however, that the very perception of pain, and hence its memory traces, are influenced by the child's interpretation of the experience. It is not really "pain" until the child, sometimes by looking at his parents and estimating their mood, decides whether he has received a spanking (been hurt) or a love-pat. Theresa Benedek discussed in some detail the child's need, upon perceiving pain, to appeal to his mother to find out whether he has been injured. She pointed out that the mother may respond to the child's need and reassure him by talking to him gently. The mother, responding to her own needs at the moment, may lose control of her own fears and express panic, or scold the child for getting hurt, adding guilt to fear—literally adding insult to injury (11). The child thus is deprived of an opportunity to observe, imitate and learn modes of behavior which he can use to increase his tolerance of anxiety and pain. He may be driven to repeat the pain in an attempt to master it and/or force magically a "better" response from his parent. In some drug dependent patients the drug represented a slightly improved version of the parent's response in regard to pain—the drug did give relief, but only postponed the anxiety *because it was itself experienced as dangerous.*

Identification and imitation of parental patterns of dealing with pain (physical and mental) are important. In some cultures patterns for dealing with pain are quite prominent.

For instance, one may be expected to drink alcohol whenever one is upset, especially during the period of mourning, to the point of complete numbing. In other cultures the noisy expression of grief and pain is encouraged and accepted both as conscious experience and as a method of dealing with the feelings involved. In yet others, the males are required to tolerate pain, grief, and so forth, stoically, without even an outward response. The patterns for handling pain and unpleasant affects are usually the same for the given culture. Pain can be a part of depression or a substitute for it (16). We have had the opportunity to observe a number of so-called iatrogenic addicts who used narcotics primarily for the relief of physical pain (e.g., headaches or abdominal pains). With remarkable consistency we found a severe latent depression warded off by massive denial, hypomanic or obsessive-compulsive mechanism. Pain, like depression or anxiety, can be the direct symptom of intersystemic intrapsychic tension.

The relationship of this formulation to the state of drug dependence is well stated by Chessick (18). The drug dependent person frequently shows little awareness of his affects. Especially in the group of "medically addicted" individuals, there is a conspicuous absence of anxiety or depression, along with a great frequency of anxiety-equivalent symptoms. In psychoanalysis or psychotherapy with narcotic and alcohol dependent persons, the discovery and verbalization of the nature of affect is an important step toward making possible the giving up of regressive symptoms.

The perception of pain, or any discomfort, tension or stimulus, is a complex process of interpretation and association. The studies by Ostow on temporal lobe function suggest that the association paths of special importance are related to memory traces of an unpleasant nature concerned with avoidance patterns (92). Perhaps this fashion of perception of pain is predestined by the anatomical structure of pain fibers in such a way that we have a quick signal at first, via the unmyelinated pain fibers, and perception of the "pain" as such arrives only some time later, permitting an evaluation of it in the meantime. Sherrington, Livingston, and others, have concluded that pain is a conscious and complex process, rather than a primary perception (64 72 79).

Physiologists have found that higher brain centers can suppress or modify the perceptual quality of pain (8 9). This seems to be the anatomical framework for the hysterical phenomena we discussed above. The time interval between the signal-perception and the full consciousness of pain can be utilized for the associative interpretation and modification of the pain experience. In the secure individual the infantile (total) fear response to pain is suppressed. This is attributable to the predominance of the secondary process, and the relatively lesser prevalence of destructive fantasies and wishes.

Inadequately understood is the mechanism by which the perception of pain is terminated psychically, as in the numbing which follows a crushing or cutting wound, or in the phenomenon of depersonalization. Our experience has been that depersonalization, *as a defense against anxiety or pain,* functions in a way exactly analogous to tissue-numbness. For instance, victims of Nazi torture very frequently became depersonalized when the torture became unbearable. Studies on convalescence by Krystal and Petty showed that either the onset of illness, development of pain, or the awareness of being ill or injured may be handled by depersonalization in normal subjects (66). One might say that either the depersonalization or the "numbing" represented a hysterical conversion symptom. Since it requires a quantity of counter-cathectic energy and ability to use it for a reversible splitting of the ego, we begin to appreciate the variety of ego functions involved in the mastery and tolerance of pain.

Of unusual research interest is the old method of managing pain by "counter-irritation." It acts as if pain tracts, a mental apparatus of perception, can be "overloaded" by other messages, such as heat or cold stimulation (from the same dermatomes), thus making the perception of pain indistinct. A host of pain relievers function on the basis of "overloading the lines" of an affected area with perception of heat, cold, sound, and so forth, thus muffling the conscious experience of pain.

Psychic pain can be handled in a similar manner. Freud has noted that counter-irritations or distractions are utilized to cope with physical and psychic pain, as in mourning. The mourner distracts himself, and only periodically returns to perceive the pain of loss, and to rework the loss piecemeal (36). The ability for such self-distraction, vis-à-vis pain of psychic or somatic origin, requires adequate energy and diversified object investments of the ego, which *clinically* can be seen to be impaired in many drug dependent persons. This is shown by the paucity and primitive nature of their object relations and gratifications. This is another mechanism involved in utilization and tolerance of pain. Tolerance for pain is a complex of ego functions which, when impaired, may create a greater than usual need of (and therefore a tendency to) drugs for the relief from pain of physical or psychic origin, in order to be able to tolerate the stresses of everyday living.

It is our contention that the very same ego-functions which are utilized in the reaction to physical pain become involved in the *handling of unpleasant (painful) affects,* and that these functions may be deficient, causing the organism to be less able to tolerate pain, anxiety, and so on, as signals. The individual who cannot deal with the unpleasant states becomes subject to stress and trauma. Szasz pointed out that anxiety is analogous in the ego-object orientation to the role of pain in self-perception in the ego-body plane of reference (114). Furthermore, there are parts of all those ego-functions which together are referred to as the "stimulus barrier." In the conscious experience of "pain," anxiety is an indispensable part of its urgent quality.

THE PROBLEM OF TRAUMA

Closely related to the subject of pain and painful affects, and perhaps even constituting only a variant of the same theme, is the concept of trauma. Freud stated that "the essence of a traumatic situation is an experience of helplessness on the part of the ego in the face of accumulation of excitation, whether of external or internal origin" (38). Dorsey indicates that the term trauma introduces an economic concept. "It means my inability to sustain and keep my mental balance when the exertion I am undergoing, the mental excitation I am suffering, is more than I can tolerate and, at the same moment, arouse my awareness for my identity" (23). The phenomenon of trauma includes "paralysing, immobilizing, or rendering to a state of helplessness, ranging from numbness to an emotional storm in affect behavior"; also "disorganization of feelings, thoughts and behavior, as well as physical symptoms reflecting autonomic dysfunction" (97). We would prefer to emphasize that this autonomic overaction is actually part of overwhelming and overflowing affect and that the affect disorganization represents a regression in which the affects are de-differentiated and discharged in a total excitation pattern like the infant. By definition, once the traumatic process is initiated, it represents a chain of unconscious reactions, which may result in a variety of specific and lasting psychopathological states. Among these, increased susceptibility to future traumatization and decreased ability to tolerate affects, and to utilize them as signals, are virtually unavoidable (109).

Raskin, Petty, and Warren related the question of trauma to drug dependence (addiction) in the following manner:

> Through every stage of the development of the addiction the person we are dealing with is helpless to make an adequate adjustment by himself. His personality is characterized by serious defects in its development and pathological tendencies inherent in its structure. He is intolerant of anxiety. He avoids or escapes experiencing it through impulsive action. Before discovering the effect of drugs, his sense of security and well-being are dependent upon the immediate gratification of his needs and wants. The ordinary delays and inconveniences of daily living are experienced by him as intolerable frustrations. He cannot escape them. Unbearable tensions are experienced which he feels the environment should relieve. When the relief is not forthcoming, he feels that his inalienable right to happiness as a human being has been abrogated. Thus, simultaneously confronted with the irresistible need for immediate gratification and an ungratifying environment, it is inevitable that he will feel justified in employing anv measure to rectify his deprivation. (101)

The drug dependent personality as such does not exist. There are a variety of factors and influences, however, which make drug use, abuse, and dependence more likely. Among the factors discussed so far, several suggest that drugs are used to avoid impending psychic trauma in circumstances which would not be potentially traumatic to other people. Such potential sources are regression vis-à-vis affect, the inability to utilize anxiety or affects as a signal, and the inability to tolerate pain and painful affects, especially the Ur-affects or predecessors of depression and anxiety. Since this Ur-affect is conceptualized as the infant's reaction to loss, it begs the question of object relations, which will be taken up later.

The point to be made is that the resistance to trauma, the stimulus barrier, is defective in drug dependent persons.

The stimulus barrier

The stimulus barrier has usually been visualized as a wall, or as Freud put it, a "crust" or "protective shield," analogous to the hornified layer of the skin:

> It acquires the shield in this way: its outmost surface ceases to have structure proper to living matter, becomes to some degree inorganic and thenceforward functions as a special envelope or membrane resistant to stimuli. In consequence, the energies of the external world are able to pass into the next underlying layers which have remained living, with only a fragment of their original intensity; and these layers can devote themselves behind the protective shield to the reception of the amounts of stimulus which have been allowed through it. By its death, the outer layer has saved all the deeper ones from a similar fate, unless, that is to say, stimuli reach it

which are so strong that they break through the protective shield. (37)

This model of the stimulus barrier, derived from the function of the skin and the sensory organs, is inadequate in that it does not acknowledge that dealing with stimuli and affects is an active process. This analogy does not view the protection of the organism against trauma as an active ego function but as a sort of sieve or dam which performs entirely passively, unselectively, and whose function is not subject to variation. We would prefer to define the stimulus barrier as the sum total of all the individual's resources which prevent or work toward the prevention of the syndrome of traumatization.

Stimulus barrier and affect tolerance

In meeting and coping with perceptions, affects, and ideas, many methods and ego functions are employed. The development of a crust might be effective in raising the stimulus threshold, but not the stimulus tolerance. Especially in relation to painful states, it is essential to distinguish between the acuity of perception of the stimulus and the affects arising from dealing with the perception. We are concerned with pain tolerance and not pain threshold. We wish to make explicit our view that the mastery of affects involves the same problems as that of external stimuli, and that the failure to master, to keep within bounds of tolerance, or to ward off affects can produce psychic trauma. Similarly, memories and unconscious memory traces pose a danger of overwhelming the ego with the intensity of stimulation related to previous perceptions (including those understood only later), memories of trauma in the past, and traumatic screens (40 97). We conceptualize the drug dependent patient's plight as living in the dread of being overwhelmed with the primary un-pleasure affects as a result of the after affects of trauma in infancy. These persons function as though they had an un-conscious memory of this danger of trauma by being over-whelmed with the Ur-affect of anxiety-depression, and must ward it off by the mechanism of denial and their dependence upon drug effects.

An interesting correlate at this point is a clinical observa-tion so frequently experienced in meeting with opiate de-pendent persons. The deficit in the integrity of their psychic stimulus barrier almost seems to be unconsciously perceived by these persons. Their inability to deal adequately and effectively with the stimulus and its provoked affectual re-sponse is eloquently expressed by their consciously stated desire and aim to gain a status of "oblivion" through the use of the drug. This same goal in relation to dealing with potential traumatizing affects is reflected by Chein (17: p. 229) in his considerations of drug dependence and Nirvana. The opiate dependent person is stated to be seeking Nirvana rather than Paradise. The latter represents an ideal situation in which all desires are easily and immediately satisfied; Nirvana constitutes the ideal of fulfillment through the absence of desire, and desire itself is viewed as an inherently frustrated state that cannot be compensated for through the pleasure of its gratification.

Use of drugs in augmenting stimulus barrier

The traumatic situation, however, is difficult to recognize because of the multiplicity of functions involved. For one, the threat is not exactly from the intensity of stimuli but, as Murphy pointed out, "the specific intensity of meaning" (84). In fact, the absence of stimuli can be just as disturbing. Also, intense stimulation or affect may be preferred, sought by drug users in warding off that which is threatening. This might be the way the amphetamine and other stimulant drug users prefer to tolerate excitement, hypomania, sensory hyperacuity, and the physiological aspects of anxiety (jitters, etc.) rather than the threatening depression or boredom. One might say that the stimulus barrier in this instance is augmented by drugs, exciting perceptions and affects against the specific threatening perception. The analogy that fits this picture better is the "living" action at cell membranes selectively absorbing some ions and using the exertion of others in the process, and at the same time the balance between the two for maintaining the pH, and the electrochemical charge at the surface—and who knows how many other functions at the same time?

Even the function of perception is subject to modification. Petrie showed that experimental subjects consistently decreased or increased the quantity of perceptions. The former also "reduced" the amount of pain they experienced, while under the same circumstances they later "augmented" it. Among the groups tested, alcoholics were consistently "average augmenters" and none were "reducers." Alcohol, aspirin, or placebos decreased the degree to which they augmented their perception, including pain (94). At the same time, we have commented on the drug dependent person's selective lack of or awareness of the one Ur-affect for the relief of which they take the drug. This is a selective "numbing" and blocking.

The ego functions that guard the integrity of the psyche

(and therefore the organism) are complex and interrelated. Keiser has pointed out:

> The loss of any one function must necessarily affect all the functions of the ego, since the ego must compensate, or find other means of satisfaction, for those drives or partial drives that can no longer be discharged or gratified through their accustomed pathways. Furthermore energy must be expended on the alteration of the ego function. Hence, it can be postulated that whenever the barrier surrounding a specific ego function is threatened with extinction, a feeling of psychic helplessness is generated. The clinical results of this feeling of helplessness may then be manifest primarily in the area of the damaged ego function. (54)

What we are observing with drug dependent individuals in regard to ego functions may have a prehistory in terms of disturbances of drives and affects (61), a resulting disturbance of the ability to deal with the affects, and consequently all the variety of abnormalities of ego functions we are describing here. Finally, as we shall discuss later, drugs themselves are used to produce yet other (temporary) changes in ego functions and consciousness as a means of dealing with or relieving the dysphoric states produced by the disturbed functions.

Case illustration

> A man dependent upon narcotics and other drugs utilized them in major part to control anxiety. Daily he would confront the excessive load of work he had arranged. He would then think that he could not possibly handle it, and this thought would further frighten him that he could not possibly face his public—hence he had to take his drug. Besides anxiety-depression, he also dreaded other affects; helplessness

drug dependence

most of all, anger, boredom, and without having been aware
of it until the analysis, sexual excitement. He managed to
avoid discovering his fear of sexual excitement because of the
use of the drugs, and before that a counterphobic promiscuity
and transvesticism.

The fear of sexual excitement was related to a childhood
strain-trauma* of a seductive older sister who, in her acting
as a substitute mother for years, used to arouse more excitement in him than he could handle. The primary trauma, however, was unsatisfactory mothering by his depressed mother.
This man lived in constant danger of return of his traumatization, now by his own affect. His experience of his affects,
especially the dysphoric ones, was that they threatened to
overwhelm him. While fearful of affects and taking drugs "for
them," after taking the drug he was able to experience the
physiological expressive parts of them, especially of anxiety,
without being panicked by the experience, and in fact with
enjoyment, betraying the erotization (deneutralization) of the
affects.

Effect of trauma on affect tolerance

This patient illustrates a disturbance in regard to the
handling of most affects, related to a dysfunction of his
maternal love objects. Boyer has pointed out that it is a part
of the maternal function to provide a barrier against en-
dogenous and exogenous stimuli for the baby, and excessive
stimulation or deprivation from the maternal love object as
well (15). The failure of this protective function would
threaten the overwhelming of the child with his affect,
threatening his survival, and interfering with his ability to
handle affects as only one of the resulting ego disturbances.

* In Kris's sense (58) it related not to a single seduction but to a con-
tinuously seductive and frustrating relationship with his sister.

Greenacre has implied that this type of maternal failure may result in the establishment of character trait disturbances and even establish the physical patterns of responses to affects; these people would be thus threatened with more violent reactions (45).

Krystal has pointed out in connection with studies of withdrawal phenomena that there is a "rebound" of the somatic aspects of affects suppressed by drugs on a subcortical level (61), and that whenever psychotropic drugs are used, some "break-through" of the expressive aspects of the drugs allows the maintenance of their effectiveness (63). The ability to alleviate some withdrawal symptoms representing a rebound of the feeling of anxiety and depression is a protection against the development of drug dependence. Conversely, an over-reactivity to these affects, and an inability to handle them in small quantities, increases the probability of addiction. In drug dependent persons there is evidence of both phenomena, and hypercathexis of those parts of the body related to affect expression—namely, the muscular and visceral organs. Chodorkoff has demonstrated corresponding changes in body-image in psychological studies of alcoholics (19 20).

We are dealing, then, with a disturbance in the handling of unpleasant affects, resulting from a failure of the protective and guiding role of the mother in providing what Winnicott called a "good enough holding environment" (118). Khan's concept of cumulative trauma fits this situation well. As he puts it, "cumulative trauma is the result of the breaches in the mother's role as a protective shield over the whole course of the child's development, from infancy to adolescence—that is to say, in all those areas of experience where the child continues to need the mother as an auxiliary ego to support his immature and unstable ego functions" (55).

While Khan discusses a variety of disturbances that result from the mother's failure to provide the shielding function as needed, he also points out that she "sponsors the capacity for toleration of tensions and unpleasure, thus promoting structural development" (55). If this process fails, and the individual has an inadequate ability to tolerate tension and unpleasant affects, the differentiation of the forerunners of these affects into depression and anxiety is impaired, the signal function of anxiety does not develop, and the threat of psychic trauma looms large through life, making the use of drugs necessary.

DRUGS AND THE PLEASURE-PAIN PRINCIPLE

In previous discussions of the ways drugs are used for relief of the unpleasant Ur-affects, we have generally referred to their blocking. We have, however, noted in one case that upon taking the drug, some somatic experiencing of the affect became possible, and was experienced with excitement and pleasure. This situation must prevail in the use of the amphetamine-like drugs, which stimulate the release of norepinephrine, and thus initiate the somatic changes of anxiety.

Thrills and regressions of affect

In the use of barbiturates, while the ideational perception of danger is minimized, it often becomes possible to experience some anxiety equivalents (e.g., heart-pounding, chills, and various skin and mucous membrane sensations), while the breathing takes on a sighing character. Thus the libidinization of anxiety may be an important aspect of some drug dependence. Some barbiturate users experience their anxiety equivalents as "thrills." The anxiety provoking experience of becoming aware of the narcotic effect of a drug is sometimes related by the patient to the return of fear first experienced while being anesthetized for a surgical procedure. The fear of "going under" may be reexperienced, even though fleetingly, while the patient is conscious of becoming sedated by, say, a sleeping pill. However, our observation of some patients, especially those who tend to develop "pathological intoxication" with alcohol or other drugs, suggests that the allegedly insensible overactivity of the anesthesiologist's "first plane of anesthesia" may, in fact, represent the expression of anxiety experienced by the partly narcotized individual in terms of loss of self-control, fear of inability to recover consciousness, or fear of death. Thus the source of "thrill" in drug use may be a source of panic, and seems to be related to the repetition compulsion.

Szasz has noted the importance of counter-phobic attitudes in addiction, as well as the importance of allowing a mastery-through-play of ambivalent object substitutes (115). This will be discussed in relation to placebo studies.

The principle of constancy

We can no longer assume that the relief from conscious anxiety provided by the drug comes only from its analgesic action directly, that is, by a chemical blockage of the function of conscious perception of intersystemic tensions. We must add to this its ability to permit regression, and thus allow discharge of impulses, affording relief in terms of the constancy principle. At other times drugs are used for the very opposite purpose—to prevent regression, as brilliantly described by Glover (42), thus avoiding this particular dread.

Studies on sensory deprivation show that a total lack of stimuli is anxiety provoking and suggest the necessity of objects for normal ego function. Pertinent here is Freud's quotation of the work of Fechner in *Beyond the Pleasure Principle:*

> Insofar as conscious impulses always have some relation to pleasure and unpleasure having a psycho-physical relation to conditions of stability and instability . . . every psycho-physical movement crossing the threshold of consciousness is attended by pleasure in proportion as, beyond a certain limit, it deviates from complete stability; while between the two limits, which may be described as qualitative thresholds of pleasure and unpleasure, there is a certain margin of aesthetic indifference. (37)

The recent work of Bowlby on mourning stresses the dependence of normal ego function on one's love objects. The *disorganization* attending the object loss and the cathectic shifts in mourning are seen as a most painful and anxiety-laden experience (14). An added dimension in the pleasure-pain series is the ego's perception of self control or organization. We believe anxiety is not caused by the pressure of undischarged drives alone, but also *involves the conception of the danger and unpleasure of disorganization.* This aspect becomes important in the consideration of schizoid personality types who seem to live in constant danger of disorganization. Many alcoholics and other drug dependent persons fall into this category. They seem to be unable to give up or change libidinal positions, but tend to try to preserve the relations in phantasy through regression.

Studies utilizing the newer drugs affecting the central nervous system (CNS) suggest that some of them depress certain brain functions while selectively stimulating others. The newer anatomical knowledge of inhibitor areas of the cortex and reticular formation gives rise to practically unlimited combinations of ways of modifying an organism's drives and their controls. The work of Olds (91), for instance, seems to be pertinent to the concept of pharmacogenic orgasm as formulated by Rado (95). On the one hand, a drug can give relief by depressing the whole brain, thus dulling all consciousness and perception. Drugs may facilitate drive expression by suppressing inhibitor areas or functions concerned with conscious self-control. Finally, drugs may cause drive discharge by the direct stimulation of appropriate brain centers.

"Corruption" of life enhancing functions of the
erotogenic zones

Olds, working with rats which had permanently implanted electrodes in their CNS that made possible electrical self-stimulation of distinct areas of the brain, showed that the animal quickly became "addicted" to self-stimulation of certain brain centers. The stimulation of "reward systems" at the midline tracts to the rhinencephalon produced an apparently pleasurable response that the animal preferred to food. It gave up all survival or sexual activities, and self-stimulated itself several thousand times a day.

When the self-stimulatory circuit was disconnected, the animal became apathetic and fell asleep (91). This recalls the effect on humans of intravenously-given opiates, especially heroin. The possibility is raised that narcotics, by a direct effect on the CNS, perhaps on specific brain centers, allow an orgasm-like discharge. This dependence upon an artificially-induced drive discharge and the consequent pharmacotoxic orgasm imply a modification of the pleasure principle, its "corruption," in the sense that it no longer serves survival or supports adaptive activity.*

Our psychoanalytic work with drug dependent individuals raises the question of the constancy principle as the exclusive principle in gratification. The idea of the accumulation of tension and its discharge in an orgasm was developed on the model of the male orgasm, and supported in observations on convulsive phenomena and some "thrills."

While the orgasm mode of discharge is one valid model, we must acknowledge another type of gratification: the relief from unpleasant stimuli or states (e.g., eating stops the tension of hunger). Satiety is pleasant in itself, but only allegedly in infants may feeding culminate in an orgasm. If the eating is pleasing, that is, stimulating by itself (*Mit dem Essen kommt der Appetit*), we are dealing with a gratification different from foreplay, as it does not lead to an orgiastic discharge. Chewing coca-leaves anesthetizes the stomach and gives gratification neurologically similar to being nourished, but certainly is different in regard to the general function and survival of the organism (70). And does not a full and digesting stomach send proprioceptive

---

* Incidentally, a similar corruption of the biological function of the pleasure principle takes place in counter-phobic reactions, in which the dominant goal is to master the anxiety at the cost of repeated exposure to danger.

signals, albeit of a different kind, just as an empty or anesthetized one does? The implications of these observations are very important to our understanding of the metapsychology of anxiety, pleasure, and the various affects in the unpleasure series as well.

The economic principle becomes involved here. To the concept of accumulation of tension from instinctual needs is added the tension produced by pain and unpleasant states, such as hunger and anger. The relief of tension, then, will be produced by a discharge of drive or relief from the painful stimulus.

The relief principle

Very pertinent here are some observations reported to the American Psychoanalytic Association Panel on Female Frigidity, 1961. Helene Deutsch, especially, made the point that the phenomenon of orgasm as patterned on the male ejaculatory and orgiastic experience (as well as phenomenological observation of infants) may not apply to the sexual function of some normal women (81). Certainly, it does not apply to the pleasure obtainable in erotogenic zones other than the genitals. This modification of our concept of gratification has important implications in our approach to drug dependent persons. It is possible that a desired endpoint of gratification is the relief or blocking of feelings of unpleasure, which may be produced not only by instinctual tensions, but also by pain, painful affects, or unpleasant states. What seems applicable here is Freud's concept of the relief principle which he described in *Beyond the Pleasure Principle,* in relation to traumatization, as "to obtain control, or bind the excitation, not in opposition to the pleasure principle but independently of it, and in part without regard to it" (37).

The function of the pleasure principle is further affected by the fact that the use of drugs prevents the drug dependent person from building up psychic tension which can be released in normal activities experienced as pleasurable. This general lowering of tension, which makes the usual pleasure discharge impossible for the drug dependent person, is another side effect of this type of self medication. With it, tension-tolerance and consciousness are also impaired.

In dealing with drug dependence, therefore, it becomes dynamically and therapeutically relevant to pinpoint the specific effect sought by the particular person. The therapist has to be aware of the specific type of relief the patient craves. The pharmacogenic effect is of no less importance than the meaning of the act to the patient in terms of its symbolic wish-fulfillment. Yet, the *meaning* to the patient of the use of the drug remains of great intrinsic importance.

II

object-representation
and self-representation

PLACEBO STUDIES

In considering the effect of drugs, we would like to isolate the effect of taking a drug from its physiological and chemical influences. We have reasons to expect that the drug represents a transference object, that it has symbolic meaning, and that the taking of the drug can serve a kind of psychic self manipulation. Placebo studies provide an excellent tool for the study of the psychological effects of taking a drug. After taking an inert medication, patients are able to produce or relieve themselves of symptoms which they could not do "on their own."

In the clinical use of opiates for analgesia, morphine relieves pain in about 75 percent of all cases. Inert placebo, given to pain sufferers of all kinds, affords relief in 35 percent of all cases (6). The placebo effect is a research tool that enables us to measure the suggestion capability of an individual vis-à-vis his pain perception. To put it differently, it gauges a person's own capacity to relieve himself of his symptoms. The placebo "reactors" produce a spectacular array of untoward reactions in from 8 to 50 percent of cases, as shown by Beecher in his summary of fifteen studies (9). As high as 10 percent of placebo reactors produce serious "toxic" reactions, such as various dermatoses, urticaria, diarrhea, and angioneurotic edema (120).

In a study of the effectiveness of an oral analgesic, placebo produced "more euphoria than did codeine" (47). A study in which placebo tablets were used as "tranquilizers" and "energizers" on the ward of a psychiatric hospital showed that from 53 to 80 percent of the patients were said to have benefited from them for an average of from 2.6 to 4.9 weeks of the six weeks they were taking them (73). In one of our own drug studies we found that the placebo relieved anxiety with success comparable to that obtained from a known tranquilizer and two different doses of a new drug which was being tested. We found no statistically significant difference in effectiveness between the four preparations in a "double-blind" study.

In another study Beecher reported a finding to which he apparently did not attribute much importance. This was that patients tend to "overreact" to the placebo, which later loses some of its effect, but "underreact" in the beginning to active pain-relievers (7). The latter suggests that the nature of the patient's transference to the physician who gives him the medication is an ambivalent one. The latent negative transference seems to negate some of the drug effect. Such reactions become especially clear in the placebo effect of surgical procedures, in which relief is obtained on the basis of a masochistic surrender to mutilation. Medical literature, as well as tradition, reminds us of the importance of the counter-transference cure in placebo action. To Sir William Osler is attributed the admonition, "One should treat as many patients as possible with a new drug while it still has power to heal." In the last analysis, however, the patient is the agent doing his own healing, "inspired" by the placebo (24). We are thus forcibly turned to the transference and therefore repressive implication of the placebo effect. In other words, the drug becomes a substitute for the love object and the yearned for type of relation with the object is ingestion and incorporation of it. Greenson has pointed out that such processes do take place universally, without the medium of a pill passed from the inspirational source to the object of enthusiasm (46). A drug, food, or even idea, in the phantasies of borrowing, acquiring or "introjecting," can be applied to relieve or counteract unpleasant states or affects. The individuals who have a tendency to drug dependence have a lower tolerance for unpleasant states. In addition, where they try to raise it by the intake of a drug, they run into difficulty because of the ambivalence towards the love object of their past, reexperienced towards the drug. Another reason these individuals cannot utilize the drugs, as do "social users" or successful addicts, is their inordinate guilt about oral indulgence, related to cannibalistic problems (41). This complication becomes especially conspicuous in the "hangover" (59), with its famous orally conceived cure referred to as "eating the hair of the dog that bit you."

THE OBJECT AND OBJECT-REPRESENTATION

Another conspicuous area of disturbed function of drug dependent persons which has been described often is their disturbed relationship to love objects (18 95 103). As part of this disturbance, they have a constant need for "external" supplies (103). The obverse side of the very same phenomenon—almost another way of stating it—is that because of a number of problems, among which are the narcissistic types of object-relation and ambivalence to them, drug and alcohol users tend to become chronically depressed. They are unable to adjust upon the loss of a love object, and develop a variety of "hangovers" of the "morning after" phenomena (59).

As will be demonstrated, there is a disturbance of the process of individuation and formation of benign self-representation and object-representation in certain types of drug dependent persons. The self-representation and the ego become impoverished and dependent upon "external" or outside supplies. A most conspicuous symptom which reflects this state, reported by Savitt (103), Chein (17), Raskin (101), and others, is the craving to gain surcease from all tension through the procurement and use of drugs. These patients express wishes and fantasies to obtain a state of Nirvana through fusion with the drug as an object substitute. They are, however, able to attain this state only momentarily, and spend all their time and effort in its ever-failing pursuit.

It is our further impression that while these drug dependent individuals yearn for a fusion with the object, they must simultaneously maintain a rigid externalization. They use the drug as a transubstantiation,* a constantly repetitive validation of the existence of the object, and the possibility of fulfillment of their fantasy of introjection.

---

* The phrase is, of course, borrowed from the Christian theological doctrine that the body and blood of Christ materialize in the sacrament of the Eucharist, and thus God can be literally ingested.

Nature of the repressed object

One additional preliminary observation involves the commonly perceived state of actual or impending clinical depression, which seems to evolve from a very characteristic ambivalence in the sphere of object-relationships. It is quite probable also that many side effects and complications of drug abuse stem from an inability of the drug dependent person to adjust to the real or fantasied loss of the love object.

By using the term "object-relationships," however, it must be acknowledged that we are indulging in a common convention. It is an inaccuracy which illustrates the repressive uses of language. As has been pointed out repeatedly by other authors (25 89), it is not with objects per se that we are concerned, but with object-representations and self-representations within the ego. Novey has discussed with great lucidity the need for clarification of this point (89). He pointed out that Sterba stressed that "the 'concept of cathexis of mental energy' applies to the object-representation, and since the 'psychic energy derives from various levels,' the object-representation is endowed with certain attributes, or experienced in ways characteristic of the conceptions of certain libidinal levels, e.g., as excrement or food" (110).

Novey also reviewed Federn's point of view on "reality perception" (31). He concluded that Federn's emphasis on the function of the ego and its boundaries permitted a "redefinition of the concept of secondary narcissism." It is to be conceptualized as dealing with distribution of energy "within the ego," so that in secondary narcissism, cathexes withdrawn from object-representations are invested in the self-representations.

Clarification of the concept of self-representation and self has been provided by Hartmann, Lowenstein and Kris (48 49), Fenichel (32), and Jacobson (51). Fenichel has pointed out the necessity to acknowledge a plurality of self-representations derived from various self-perceptions of our mental or bodily states, activities or characteristics. The self-representation is further influenced by infantile fluctuations in the ability to maintain the separation from the object-representation, and the identifications or displacement of various characteristics of the object-representations to it (51). Important in the establishment of integrity and maturity of self-representations is the feeling of ego identity, described by Erickson as "the awareness of the fact that there is a self-sameness and continuity to the ego's synthesizing methods" (29).

Edith Jacobson has developed in detail the multiple influences in the formation of the object-representation (51). We wish to stress with her that object-representations are also exposed to many influences and modifications. Among the early vicissitudes of object-representations, it would seem that three are most pertinent to our clinical material:

(1) *Oscillations between fusion and diffusion of self-representations and object-representations.* It has been pointed out that after the establishment of the awareness of the object-representation, there are occasions for fusion of the self-representation, especially following gratification. We can surmise that it happens also in longing for gratification through a *regression to a pre-object state.* Gradually there is an individuation and separation while

> libido and aggression are continuously turned from love
> objects to the self, and vice versa, or also from one object to
> the other, while self and object images of different objects
> undergo temporary fusion and separate and join again. Simul-
> taneously, there is a tendency to cathect one such composite
> image with libido, while all the aggression is directed to
> another until ambivalence can be tolerated. (51)

(2) The object-representations are cathected with the
libido of the currently predominant partial drives, and experienced accordingly, as "food to be ingested, or feces to
be excreted," and so on. This issue will be especially pertinent to the nature of the object-representations in drug
dependent individuals who experience their object in a
narcissistic (need supplying) and oral (to be ingested)
frame of mind.

(3) *Problems of ambivalence, and more specifically,
aggression in early object-representation.* Jacobson's comments on the work of Melanie Klein were basically in the
line of correcting the usage of the words "introjection,"
"projection," etc., in terms of the relations of the object-
representation and self-representation (51 56). Her points
seem to be quite helpful. Obviously, not the object but the
object-representation is "introjected." Not the self but the
self-representation or ego seems to "fall to bits" when threatened by aggressive impulses. On the other hand, Jacobson
rejects the importance of the effect of the infant's dread of
his aggression. Experienced magically and omnipotently, it
may seem to threaten the "destruction of the world." In fact,
the world destruction fantasies in the schizophrenic are a
reference to such fears, though not an accurate regression,
because in the meantime many changes have taken place
in one's image of the self and world. In drug dependent

persons, oral characters in general, the history of oral frustration and rejection in infancy is common (95 103). Under these circumstances, aggression directed toward the mother or self seem to be experienced as life-threatening. It seems to require massive repression, with a resulting permanent effect upon the individual's character and the nature of his handling of the object-representations. This point will be elaborated upon later, inasmuch as it constitutes an essential element of the thesis of this presentation. But before discussing the results of the particular handling of aggression in our drug dependent patients, let us first observe their clinical characteristics as compared to depressive and schizophrenic patients.

OBJECT-REPRESENTATION AND SELF-REPRESENTATION IN DEPRESSION

In states of depression, as in the state of mourning, there is a notable ambivalence towards the lost love object. Depressed persons often become involved in pathological mourning, and sometimes it becomes apparent that the depression is the result of a fall in self-esteem accompanied by reproaches toward the self displaced from the object. This has been described by Freud and Fenichel: "By virtue of introjection, a part of the patient's ego has become the object" (32). "The shadow of the object has fallen on the ego" (36).

In mourning, the object-representation forcibly returns to demonstrate its nature as the product and part of one's mental life. The loss of one's real love object only adds to the attributes of the object-representation. It does not make the object-representation disappear. Mourning represents a time for the correcting of mental bookkeeping, a time of elaboration of our relations with our object-representations. Under normal circumstances one can go a step beyond the formation of clearly distinct self-representation and object-representation. With increased insight, and through what Wetmore calls "effective grieving" or its equivalent in analysis (117), one can usually extend the boundaries of his consciously perceived selfness to include his lost object-representations. There are obvious advantages to being able to recognize that one can deal only with his own mental representation of his love objects. Such expansion in the quality of selfness, however, may evoke fear (e.g., a man with poor masculine identity and fear of homosexual impulses may be frightened to recognize that so far as he is concerned he has to create and mentally *be* his own wife).

We feel that the failure to own up to the self-sameness of one's own mental material, whether self, object or environmental representation, is a most prevalent form of repression. In fact, overcoming the repressive use of language, and the various subtle ways of repression of one's own living and mental material, would represent a difference as marked as between the primary and secondary process. Accordingly, the term "tertiary process" has been suggested to describe this additional extension and integration of cognition and reflective awareness. Dorsey, who coined this phrase, has contributed his thoughts on its meaning for this occasion:

> My continuing self analysis, in that it consists of investing my mind with consciousness for the truth that it is *my* mind that I am using, ultimately results in my extending my ac-

knowledgeable personal identity to include all of my self experience.

Every other kind of psychogenesis with the exception of this specific process of enlightening my mentality with *appreciation* for its being mine, involves the development of unconscious mentality.

Thus, the primary process may involve no self insight, or conscious self identity. However, the secondary process does entail the investment of mental events with consciousness that may or may not be recognized as consisting of nothing but self identity (despite the fact that Sigmund Freud pointed out there can be no consciousness but self consciousness). Functioning of the powers of the secondary process may be, and seemingly mostly is, experienced without the featuring of the truth that all of it is entirely and only self activity. Therefore, the need for a category of psychic activity solely and wholly serving acknowledgeable truth of *responsible* self consciousness is evident. On account of its great benefit to me I have dignified this process of awakening to my true self identity in all of my living with the term: tertiary process.

I see that I have no choice as to whether I shall be an absolute solipsist or not, for as an absolute individual, solipsism is all that is possible for me. The only possible choice I have in this matter is whether or not I shall consciously acknowledge and assert my necessary solipsistic individuality.

The impoverishment of the ego of the drug dependent person shows a paucity of self-sufficiency feelings. (25)

It is usually a comfort to the mourner to realize that the "deceased will live on in our midst." As a matter of fact, the Jewish religion originally used this idea, instead of the concept of the hereafter, for the denial of death. Ahad Ha-Am pointed out that in Jewish theology life was considered to be continued within the community by being "passed on." Life going on within the community was symbolized by giving the names of the deceased to the newborn (12). But as we all know, the aggression towards the object-representation makes the fantasy of introjection of the object into the self-representation dangerous, and contributes to the creation of the problems of depression after the loss of the object. Some of the pain in mourning and depression, especially the part caused by self-reproaches, is related to the return of repressed and (internally) projected aggression on to the object-representation. The ability to keep the object-representation separate from the self-representation is one way to deal with one's aggression, at least temporarily. The separateness of the object-representation protects one's self-representation from becoming flooded with aggression.

In mourning there is a "penetration" of the borders of self-representation by the object-representation which now returns from repression-by-alienation. This is experienced as pain. This is analogous to Freud's concept of physical pain as the mental representation of the penetration of the frontiers of our physical integrity. The pain is proportional to the urgency to repress aggression and to encapsulate and wall off the object-representation. This defense is motivated by the dread of destructive impulses toward the love object. To avoid pain, only the "good" part of the object-representation may be "introjected" into the self-representation, while the "bad" part of the ambivalently loved object-representation is exiled as a demon, ghost, or the like (35). In depression, the bad part is attributed to the self-representation.

Object-representation in schizophrenia

Bak has pointed out that in the schizophrenic the fusion between the self-representation and the object-representation is utilized as a specific defense against aggression directed against the object-representation (4). Under such circumstances, we observe regression to a "pre-object-representation separation" state. Nacht and Viderman have pointed out that some patients are unable ("refuse") to accept a dyadic relationship, which is experienced by them as too painful or threatening because of a "renewed separation and fresh wound."

> We sometimes reach a deeper, more secret and unchanging level of psychic structure characterized by an intense need for absolute union, at which the individual appears to desire nothing better than a return to the original world in which there was, as yet, no separation. (87)

Under these circumstances, delusional transference "fusion" with the therapist may occur, such as described by Margaret Little. Working with borderline personalities, she found that their

> "basic fault" is a failure of differentiation and integration, splitting being an ego activity belonging to a later stage of development. Borderline . . . people . . . cannot in any circumstance take survival for granted. There exists in their memories a representation of something which we must really regard as annihilation. The idea is that a basic feeling of unity between baby and mother is a protection against this dread . . . they tend to form a delusional transference of total identity with the analyst . . . a state of total undifferentiation I have called "basic unity." (71)

A common occurrence in the treatment of schizophrenic patients in the development of transference fantasies of fusion with the therapist is total identity with him. In borderline cases, also, are encountered fantasies of fusion with God (e.g., of "oceanic" type) or with the transcendental. This type of transference is based on the idealization of the object and simultaneous vilification of the self-representation. However, in the treatment of alcohol or drug patients, we have only rarely observed this type of transference. These patients are involved in a struggle against accepting the image of themselves as bad. They experience tremendous guilt after indulgence or misbehavior, but immediately come up with resolutions to become "perfect" tomorrow. We believe that in drug dependence permanent fusion is not possible because of the nature of the fantasies.

We have frequently observed and previously reported that they do much better when treated in a clinic facility where they can "split up" the transference and experience various aspects of the object-representations among a number of different members of the therapeutic team (76). Krystal has further pointed out that under these circumstances a major psychotherapeutic task is to have the "chief therapist" on a given case collect all the information of the nature of the transference resistances, acted out or expressed toward all the assistant therapists, and consider them as being directed toward him. Interpretations which bring together the fragmented transferences may be used by the patient to form unified object-representations through work analogous to grieving (62). Although yearned for, a permanent fusion of the self-representation with the object-representation is impossible, and the acceptance of a temporary, failing but renewable, substitute is accepted. In the course of developing the drug dependence, the act of taking the drug, the drama of its effect and its losing its effect, and even the withdrawal, all become hypercathected with libidinal and aggressive energy. This is one of the reasons why only short-acting drugs are satisfactory for drug dependent persons, despite their loud protestations to the contrary.

In fact, one is inclined to speculate whether the psychoses and panic "bad trips" after LSD and other long-acting drugs are not related to the enforced feeling of drug effect for a long time. It may be precisely because the fantasy of fusion with the object is both yearned for and dreaded that it can be tolerated only in readily terminable doses.

RÉSUMÉ OF OBJECT-REPRESENTATION IN DRUG DEPENDENCE

Alcoholic, narcotic, barbiturate, and other drug-dependent persons are not noted for their ability to relate to "real" objects. People and objects external to themselves are but sources and providers of supplies which can be "taken in." Their need is to find object-substitutes which produce a status of infantile satiation-fusion (95 103). This bliss, though, lasts only a short time and then new supplies have to be ingested. The much desired fulfillment of the ingestions—introjections of the object—repeatedly fails. Why is this craved fusion between the self-representation and the object-representation, which is so singularly impossible, pursued with such an overwhelming compulsion? Some illustrative case material may be helpful:

Case illustrations

(1) A fairly young alcoholic woman described in the course of an hour that she was quite tired and "perhaps depressed."

She felt that her tiredness might be due to the way she felt driven to work all day long. In the morning she spent most of her time playing with her little girl till noontime, when she would take her to kindergarten. She felt compelled to do this to ensure that her daughter was not "left alone" as she herself had been. She was the firstborn child in her parents' home. Her mother had repeatedly told her that her parents were "not ready" for her, and her father so resented her that he never did soften in his rejection of her. When she was less than two years old, her younger sister was born, whom the patient never got along with. At present a serious marital crisis was "caused" by the patient's feeling that her husband was too devoted to and spent too much time with his mother. She was also depressed "because" her period was due the next day. She was "always" depressed before and during her menses. She had been trying to get pregnant for a few years but could not conceive.

She had a dream about her cat, which seemed to be trying to eat, but the food became spoiled and "crawled with maggots" and "other horrible worms"; later it seemed that the cat had kittens but they became very tiny and "shrunk into little lumps."

Among her associations, the patient described that since she had stopped drinking (about a month previously, when she started taking Antabuse), she discovered she had trouble sleeping. Sometimes when her husband would fall off to sleep, she would get up and have a glass of milk, or do something like "make up the grocery list." Her cat had been sprayed. Recently her little girl had treated it roughly, and as usual, the patient had difficulty reprimanding her. The daughter had brought home a toy which the patient thought she took without permission. She kept telling the child to take it back, but as she was yelling about it, her daughter got undressed and was ready for the bath, so the mother "gave up." She is always worried about food getting spoiled, and dislikes insects—any "crawly" thing.

She then talked at great length about her desire for and inability to have another child, finally realizing she was treating her daughter as she would have liked to be treated herself, feeling she was never given the love or attention she needed.

As she talked about this theme, her eyes filled and tears rolled down her cheeks, but she denied "feeling sad." Similarly, when she first came in, she said she was "fine," only gradually discovering she was depressed. The picture of the cat having kittens then led to a number of memories about "home on the farm" when kittens were drowned, and seeing her father chopping off the heads of chickens with a hatchet. She then recalled that her mother had told her she had been a "good little girl" and always played by herself or sat still "watching" while her mother took care of the baby.

This patient was married twice; the first time to an alcoholic, the second time to a very rigid, ungiving husband. She recalled that she had had intercourse in the interval since the last appointment. Her husband complained that after intercourse she was wide awake and wanted to do something or eat something instead of going to sleep. It became apparent in the course of her description that she experienced intercourse as a fulfillment of her yearning to be "united" physically with her husband. The cessation of intercourse was experienced by her as a separation, to which she responded with anxiety and agitation. One of the manifestations of the yearning to become "united" with her mate was her refusal to use rubber contraceptive devices because they interfered with her image of physical union during intercourse. This yearning always ended in the feeling of frustration. During the postcoital frustrated excitement, she started to drink wine for a "nightcap," and later also to relieve her boredom and loneliness, finally developing a drug dependence.

(2) A middle-aged alcoholic male patient opened the analytic hour with a statement that he had been feeling all right in the preceding half hour and was reluctant to disturb this condition by the analytic work. He then reported a dream he had that morning just before he woke up: a woman with whom he had once had an affair threw a bottle of acid at his wife, injuring and burning her severely. The patient reported

that in the last few days he got along a little better with his wife, so that she even called him "honey" on occasion. Over the weekend he felt "horney." However, he did not want to approach his wife for fear that she would refuse him intercourse, or do it mechanically just to please him. Instead he masturbated with fantasies about another woman with whom he had had an affair. The fantasy was entirely about fondling and sucking her breast. She had "beautiful, large breasts," in contrast to his wife, whose breasts were so small they were "almost non-existent." On inquiry about his reluctance to approach his wife, he indicated that they had had no intercourse in over a month, and then it was "just sex." He felt that he was repulsive to his wife because of being "fat." He also felt guilty that he had some drinks on weekend evenings, a habit which he has been trying to give up because of the danger of a relapse of his drinking problem.

Having considerable sophistication in working with his mental material, this being an advanced stage of his analysis, he observed that without giving his wife a chance to be nice to him, he set up a situation in which he felt justified in feeling deprived by her and giving vent to his tremendous, pent-up, ever-frightening aggression. We reviewed a number of situations where he arranged similar constellations, including acting out in the transference. He then recalled that as a child he was told that he never defied authority, but he had a recollection of being terribly angry and forcibly restrained until he was exhausted. His history was one of repeated disappointment in his wife and other love objects, by and large engineered by the patient. He similarly felt the constant dread that people in his profession and church would dislike him, but at the same time was driven to antagonize them, or to act out his fantasy of sucking out all the strength and outshining the "other guys." Recently, such acting out had almost caused the psychoanalysis to come to an abrupt end—under circumstances where he could have told himself that he was "rejected" by the analyst. Frightened by his oral aggression, he switched to the anal ideation, inquiring what could he do to "get rid" of that terrible rage and greed within him.

The patient's next analytic hour was to be early in the morning. He called about a half hour before his appointment time, telling his analyst "he could relax" because he could not come for the hour but was willing to pay for it. He explained that he was terribly involved in finishing a project which would demonstrate what a splendid job he had done for his employer. When questioned why this project could not wait for an hour, he insisted that it was too late already, and that he was so "excited and wrapped up" in his work that he just could not get his mind off it and do analytic work.

He came in the next day and made two comments: (1) prior to this hour, as he got up and was sitting on the toilet, it occurred to him that the thing he dreaded most was loneliness; (2) it then occurred to him that to him the feeling of loneliness was "the same as hunger." He associated to this that though he is basically intellectually an atheist, emotionally he has not been able to accept the idea of there being "nothing," because it is too terrifying to him in terms of the threat of loneliness and his "terror of chaos."

He then said that the analyst's inquiring why he could not get down to that project *after* the hour made him realize that he had been terribly excited about getting to work on the previous morning's project—he could hardly even stand going to sleep for the night, he was so eager to get to work on his project. However, the inquiry completely spoiled it for him and he spent a day of "torture and misery." He realized that he was again laboring under a compulsion. In the course of the hour it became apparent that (1) he constantly vacillated between the feeling of severe depression when he felt he was "ugly" and unlovable, and altogether repulsive (to him, being hungry and being ugly were one and the same thing, and ugly meant physical ugliness as well as the "uglies" of rage and greed), and (2) he distorted the nature of his object-relations because of his needs, e.g., when he does not work hard at his office he becomes terribly upset that his secretary will observe this and become critical of him. Similarly, he thought that the analyst disapproved of him when he cancelled the hour, and this thought threw him into despair.

This man was in a hypomanic excited state when he felt that his present work would bring him the long yearned for love of his parents—especially his extremely successful and unaffectionate father.

In the course of the hour it became obvious that to this patient maintaining his object-representation *outside* of himself was the prime struggle in his life, in fact the nuclear conflict. He was driven to constantly "test" the object, and to provoke it to the very limit, in order to find proof that he is still acceptable. He then talked about the fact that when he said he was starved, he did not mean food alone—because "even with Purina Dog Chow, you have to add love"—was the ingredient he had missed. He puzzled over the fact, why did he feel that if he was unloved and hungry, he was ugly and bad.

The analyst then interpreted this acting out as a repetition of his childhood handling of aggression by turning it against himself. As a result, his mother continued to be omnipotent and benevolent, but he assumed all the guilt, resulting in his seeing himself as bad, ugly and unlovable. This interpretation produced an intense emotional reaction in the patient. He started shaking his head, nodding yes and no at the same time. He then broke out in hysterical laughter, which gradually turned into sobbing. He finally was able to say, between sobs, that he wished he could deny the "crazy things" he just heard, but unfortunately he "knew in his heart" that this was exactly what happened to him. He then produced some memories which had never been available before, which showed that his mother was so depressed after his birth that an aunt was eventually brought into the house to take over the role of the mother, but "alas, too late for him."

In the patient's next analytic hour he was able to verbalize the feelings related to his past drinking pattern, and currently relived yearnings. His strongest yearning for alcohol came as a "reward" for work done or "good behavior." He seemed to need to structure the world as based on awards and praise for good deeds and achievements. However, it quickly became apparent that this model of the world was a defense against an earlier one. Most of his day was filled with dread of the next "thing," whether job or person. Associations led to the basic insecurity which he had, and terror—recalling the child breaking out in tears on seeing a stranger's face. In the patient's life, the over-reacting to danger referred to the events of the first year of his life, which he could not get over. Daily, and many times through the day, he relived the drama of terror over the helplessness and worthlessness of his self, and the expectation of reunion and introjection of the relief-giving drug or other object-substitutes.

These patients demonstrate a tendency toward repression of their object-representations by externalization. We are considering repression here to refer not only to parts of one's self-representation rendered totally unconscious, but also to various degrees of unconsciousness, including parts of one's mental material alienated by virtue of depriving it of the sense of identity.

REVIEW OF THE CONCEPT OF REPRESSION

Repression, says Dorsey, is "ignoring and denying part of one's human nature, in which he cannot see his identity with composure." It is "denying the propriety of existence of certain personal living," comparing it with renunciation, defined as "fully acknowledging the wonderfulness of certain personal living and freely allowing or restraining one's indulging it." Stating it in another way, to repress is to "repudiate one's mental material under the guise that it is some other kind of material." Dorsey addresses himself specifically to the way object-representations are handled:

To secure mind-help via mind-denial (repression) . . . First of all, it is most practical to be able to see the true nature of that which is undergoing repression, namely, one's own human nature. Unhappy "mother" or "father" or "sibling" meaning is sometimes called the "repressed mental content." Only the meaning of an individual's very own personal living can exist for him. The fact is, and needs to be said over and over, only one kind of living *can* be repressed—namely, *selfness,* the meaning constituting the personal mind of one's own individuality. (25)

This conception of repression is more in keeping with the structural theory. What is repressed and becomes unconscious is the aggression towards the object-representation and its nature as the subject's mental mechanism. The powerful counter-cathexes then cause a rigidity in the externalization of the object-representation and make its energy and modes of action unavailable to the ego. Arlow and Brenner pointed out:

It is the intensity of counter-cathexis against the psyche element in question which is important. We know from experience that only when a defense is less intense is there a chance that on interpretation to the patient of what it is that he is defending himself against can it be assimilated or integrated with the normal or healthy part of the patient's ego. (3)

In the psychic economy of a certain group of drug dependent patients there is a great feeling of impoverishment of the self-representation. The self is experienced as very weak or helpless, bad or worthless. Because of this self-image, there is a great pressure toward the fusion of self-representation and object-representation. The nature of the fantasies involved impose certain conditions and create problems in the fulfillment of this yearning:

(1) It must be an action undertaken by the object-representation's present transference "materialization." This is felt absolutely necessary because the patients have overwhelming guilt over their oral and cannibalistic strivings, so that only if the object of transference offers the love and gratification of which they feel they have been deprived, can they accept it (104).

(2) Because of the ambivalence and incorporative yearnings towards the object-representation, the patient lives in danger of throwing himself back into an overwhelming depression if such fusion does take place. In fact, it would seem that this eventuality is so dreaded that mourning becomes impossible. To illustrate:

> A young woman with a problem of alcoholism and barbiturate dependence revealed that since the death of her mother she has kept house in such a way that all appearances of the mother's presence were maintained. Her mother's little notes to her, which she had been in the habit of writing, were pinned all over the house. The patient acted in every way as though her mother was still alive. Three other observations were made: (1) one year before the mother's death, the patient's pet dog died, and in relationship to the animal, too, the patient kept denying its death completely; (2) she never dared or allowed the analyst to say or allude to the fact that her mother was dead; and (3) she entered into a love affair with a man with whom she structured the situation so that he mothered her. For instance, after they made love he would tuck her in bed and stay with her, and only *after* she fell asleep would he leave.
>
> In general, the patient tried to preserve the whole life pattern exactly as she had with her mother's presence. All this

failed, however, with outbreaks of severe depression, and with suicide attempts with an overdose of barbiturates.

To accomplish the work of mourning would be too dangerous because this type of patient has a need to keep the object-representation rigidly separated from his self-representation. There is also frequently a similar reaction to the superego, which is rigid and punitive. Hence, the need to externalize the superego and particularly to "seduce" the therapist (and before that friends and relatives) to act as an "external" superego. The rigid isolation of the superego through externalization serves to avoid painful living, at least self-consciously. The price to be paid, though, is the impoverishment of one's mental resources.

THE HANDLING OF AGGRESSION AND ITS EFFECT ON SELF-REPRESENTATION AND OBJECT-REPRESENTATION

In individuals dependent on alcohol and other drugs, *the threat of the loss of the love object is experienced as equivalent to annihilation.* The early love objects appear to have been experienced as frustrating or too seductive, and therefore very ambivalently. Aggression had to become rigidly repressed. The special tenacity of denial in the alcoholic often appears to buttress repression of this troublesome aspect of the infantile object-representation relationship.

It would seem that the problem of dealing with aggression in infancy is of crucial importance to our thesis. The child experiences his aggression as dangerous to whatever conception he has of himself and his object-world. Repression and counter-cathexes of aggressive impulses make the separation of object-representation from the self-representation pathologically inflexible. In this act, drive energy is not neutralized but repressed and requires constant energy exertion against the return of the repressed. Having repressed his mother by denying his own responsibility for creating and living her image in his own mind, he also repressed his mother's child. Parts of his own mind are walled off by counter-cathectic energy and are not available to his ego. Modes of action and thinking become reserved for the mother-image and prohibited to the child. Having eliminated the healing, sustaining mother from his self-identity, he loses a vital share of his resources for sustaining healing and comforting, acknowledging and accepting himself. Having repressed his father-image, he loses access to his aggressive, self-assertive masculinity. When an attempt is made to assume adult functions, the patient must deal with a gnawing sense of guilt and an expectation of punishment and disaster. Thus, everyday life becomes excessively painful to him. Any stressful experience becomes a major crisis of impending disaster.

Such externalization also necessitates a concrete demonstration of good will by the alienated object-representations. In a number of cases, overt suicide attempts or "accidental" overdosage to the point of coma had the latent meaning of testing whether the patient still deserved to live. Some drug dependent individuals are driven to put their lives "on the line" in arranging a concrete demonstration of the love-object-representation's life-sustaining attitude.

Being unable to achieve a fantasy fusion between his self-representation and his benign object-representation, this type of drug dependent patient is thus caught in a double bind. There is constant disappointment with the object-representation. It fails to fulfill the yearnings for fusion and Nirvana of the patient, but at the same time he must cling to the object and cannot tolerate separation. The result is the need for the repetition of the introjection of the transubstantiation of the object. The following is an autobiographical note supplied by the poet Allen Ginsberg. He describes that he was able, *without drugs,* to achieve a state of "spiritual communication" with the poet William Blake, and subsequently he experienced

> a moment of guilelessness about the world around me and feeling that the father of the universe loved me and I was identical with the father. So this was an experience of bliss. I realized that I had my place in the universe. (1)

However, later he lost this feeling, but discovered he could produce it repeatedly by taking LSD. The mystery is this:

If Mr Ginsberg is capable of reaching this ecstasy and union with God (father-mother-universe) on his own, why should he want to use a drug, thus depriving himself of the credit for such an achievement? And, once having achieved the union with God and having found his place in the universe, why does he lose it and have to go through this experience over and over again? Mr Ginsberg implies that one disadvantage of experiencing such oceanic union spontaneously is that people might consider him mad under these circumstances, but not when it is drug induced. But it appears that he also does not dare to admit to himself that he has the ability and the power to reach this "alien" part of himself, which he calls his "God and father," and has the need to terminate it promptly. Moreover, he has the need to reexperience this reunion because apparently, whether drug induced or reached by inspiration or lifting of repression, he is driven to quickly reestablish this "wall" within his mind.

In some drug dependent individuals we witness the twin phenomena of the craving for reunion and the need for separation. Upon separation, the drug wearing off, there is some experience of the Ur-affects of unpleasure, which represent the acting out, under the sway of the repetition compulsion, of the nearly deadly disappointment with the love object in infancy. This drama must be repeated, but cannot be solved. Mired down in such a state of helplessness, the drug dependent person must utilize the narcissistic, orally cathected nature of the object-representation. This makes it possible for him to substantiate a "thing" for a person and to keep using these in alternation (32). Thus, he denies the disappointment and rage toward his depriving object-representation, declaring instead that it was not the real article. Once he finds the drug, he has the "perfect" substitute, one that he can control, repeatedly introject, and that eliminates the danger of destruction of the object (46 100). It is a concrete, easily controlled source of gratification, which takes the place of human love objects, and is unconsciously experienced as the transubstantiation of the original love object.

SUMMARY

We have reviewed the vicissitudes of object-representation in the drug dependent person. We have considered the fate of the ego affected by ambivalence to the object-representation in which the aggression seems to magically threaten the destruction of the object-representation and/or self-representation. Under these conditions the object-representation becomes rigidly isolated from the self-representation by the repression of one's perception of his own aggression and the need for love and forgiveness. The ego becomes split-up in the process of denying the self-sameness of one's object-representation as a product of one's own mind and living. The ego, thus impoverished, indulges in delusional attempts toward repair and self-sustenance by the taking in of "concrete" object-substitutes which are experienced as the transubstantiation of the object. The object-substitutes, dependence producing drugs, and object-relations become endowed with ambivalent transferences and must fail just as the original object (mother) was experienced as failing during the crucial stage in the patient's life. We view drug dependence, with Dorsey (27), as an instance of extreme form of transference.

III
dealing with emotions by modification of consciousness

The manner in which drugs can be used for obtaining relief from pain, unpleasant or painful affects, has been shown to be complex. Drugs can be active in various points of the chain of mental events that produce affects. We will review and study the aspects of consciousness, ideation, self-perception, interpretation of perception and body image, and functions which are commonly modified for this purpose. The major steps in the generation of affect—the underlying conflict, the meaning and physiological (expressive) part—can all be expected to be modifiable by drugs.

We have already noted that there is a large group of individuals given to drug abuse who do so, to an important extent, for relief from unpleasant affects. They fend off this danger by a sort of "shunt" composed of an absence of conscious awareness of the affects, and take the drug at this point before they can be conscious of anxiety, depression, boredom, and/or other unpleasant states quite painful to them. While their defense against affects precludes a conscious recognition of them, some of these patients discover that their life is unhappy and devoid of pleasure or, as Dorsey's patient said, "I am two double shots behind the rest of the world" (27).

The impairment of appreciation of the behavioral and emotional changes which ensue from prolonged drug use is one of the ubiquitous problems in drug dependence. The problem is compounded by the fact that drug dependent people have an impairment of self-perception and evaluation even prior to resorting to dulling themselves with chemicals. For this reason, studies of the effect of drugs on affects are very difficult and unreliable. At least portions of such studies depend on the patients' insights, evaluations, and descriptions of their states, but they make very unsatisfactory research subjects. One recent study, though carefully planned and conceived, utilized the patient's self-rating as the primary tool in evaluating the effect of alcohol. Mayfield and Allen, in a study of the effect of alcohol on alcoholics, utilized the Clyde-Mood scale, a self-inventory involving sorting 133 adjectives in four categories of applicability. Three groups were used, alcoholics, depressives, and controls, the latter consisting of nonprofessional hospital staff. They were given intravenous alcohol. The findings were:

"The pre-fusion scores of the depressed patients indicated a pervasive and profound disturbance in affect, while the controls and alcoholic groups differed only in the jittery factor." These observations did "reflect the clinical picture of the three groups." "The depressed patients improved dramatically with intoxications; the controls showed significantly less but still definite improvement; and the alcoholics tended to improve least, and indeed showed a trend toward deterioration. These differences were also apparent in our observation of the subjects at the time of infusion" (78).

Implied in this report is the judgment that the "deterioration in function," which consisted in the alcoholic's becoming worse "on the clear thinking and energic scale," was the result of alcoholism itself and disproved the "effectiveness" of alcohol. However, we would question whether the impairment in clear thinking is *not the very effect* sought by the alcoholic. It is possible to achieve the final goal of effect blocking, modification, or reversal (to its opposite) by influencing one's cognition, judgment, or other aspects of ego function or consciousness. This point is discussed later in greater detail, after we review the relationship of consciousness to affects.

ALTERED STATES OF CONSCIOUSNESS

Ludwig has collated the common characteristics of "Altered States of Consciousness." A change in the state of consciousness can be caused by various factors such as sensory deprivation, overstimulation, ecstatic states, hypnotic and toxic states (74). Utilizing Ludwig's compilation, we find the following alterations of functions are most pertinent to our interest in affect control:

(1) Alterations in thinking with "disturbance in concentration, attention and judgment," primary process cognition, loss of reflective self-awareness and appreciation of cause-and-effect. This change lends itself to a modification in the interpretation of reality and one's psychic conflict in the direction of avoiding painful conclusions.

(2) Disturbed time sense, permitting the escape of the immediacy of unpleasant affect, and the enjoyment of a feeling of timelessness of ecstatic states.

(3) Loss of control, complete helplessness, conducive

to feelings of surrender and oceanic fusion with deified objects, in turn allowing an escape from intersystemic tensions.

(4) Changes in emotional expressiveness, with either an increased intensity in emotional expression, or a detachment and indifference to feelings experienced. This "crying in one's beer" reaction allows the expression of affect without the fear of it.

(5) Body image change, varying from depersonalization, detachment from one's body, or modifications of perception of the body as weightless, shrunken, or enlarged. The loss of the feeling of the limits of one's mind and body can be utilized in mystical and transcendental phantasies.

(6) Perceptual distortions; those used for hallucinatory wish fulfillment and need for punishment may break through.

(7) Change in meaning and significance. This feature of the states of altered consciousness, which is secondary to the change in cognition, is of special relevance to our consideration of affects, and has been singled out by Ludwig as the feeling of "profound insight, illumination and truth." He states that in toxic or psychotic states, there is an increased sense of significance to external cues, ideas of reference, and numerous instances of "psychotic insight." There is a modification in cognition, accompanied by a modification in perception, and interpretations are made under the domination of the pleasure principle. Thus the conclusions and awareness are so "edited" that no painful or unpleasant affects need develop. Perhaps the similarity is by analogy only, but the reaction to ideas here resembles the wish-directed thinking characteristic of certain brain

syndromes, such as Korsakoff's. Rapaport has described this state as a "unilinearity of consciousness" dominated by a wish (99). Wishes and ideas which become conscious as a result of being wish-fulfilling are not subjected to a critical or judgmental evaluation. Ideas which might create conflicts, self-criticism or recognition of impairment of one's function, are repressed. The most characteristic and ubiquitous result of chronic drug use is a change in the behavior pattern of which the user has no insight. The changes in some cases (especially in alcoholics or users of synthetic "non-narcotic" pain relievers) are very insidious and slowly developing, and may be difficult to define (e. g., irritability, defensiveness, greater impulsivity, or failure to respond to emergencies). But even where the changes become quite obvious, the user is the last one to know. Among the reasons for this is his need to avoid the painful affect which would develop upon this type of self-evaluation.

(8) Sense of the ineffable, that is, of having an indescribable experience of a kind that transcends the usual or ordinary. This is a specific antidote, the opposite feeling to boredom and depression.

(9) Feeling of rejuvenation, which Ludwig describes as "a new sense of hope, renaissance or rebirth." This experience is so close to the deepest hopes of a depressive person that once experienced it would likely be sought out intensely. This type of feeling experienced as part of the disturbance consciousness, by either drug inducement, comatherapy, suggestion or sleep, may start a change from a hopeless depressive to a hopefully excited (manic) affect, illustrating a type of "reversal" of affect.

(10) Hypersuggestibility, in which Ludwig includes not only susceptibility to uncritical acceptance of commands and impulses, but also the "increased tendency of a person to misperceive or misinterpret various stimuli or situations based either on his inner fears or wishes." With the dominance of the pleasure principle, the loss of the self-evaluative and critical function, it becomes possible to reinterpret every bit of mental data in a wishful way. It thus becomes possible to achieve an affect reversal or modification based on a new interpretation of the psychic reality. Even the paranoid patient (e.g., in alcoholic hallucinosis) is acting on behest of this regressed type of homeostasis, under the dominance of the pleasure ego, projecting his anxiety to the "outside." As long as this defense is successful, the anxiety can be prevented from developing by the avoidance of the object of projection.

In the production of affect, we need to consider not just the state of consciousness alone, but also some ego functions. In the summarization by Ludwig, many of these functions were referred to, such as reality testing, especially the matters of self- and body-image, the ability to maintain thinking on a verbal and predominantly secondary process level, and the degree of reflective self-awareness, to use Rapaport's term. It is useful to recall Rapaport's description of consciousness from the psychodynamic view.

> Psychoanalytic theory considers consciousness one of the means of human adaptation to reality. It considers consciousness a function of the ego, or if you prefer, an apparatus in service of the ego . . . consciousness is somehow a superordinate sense organ; what happens on the receptors, and much of what happens intraphysically, is relayed to it and represented by a certain code. (99)

Consciousness is not a quality to be perceived as an either-or phenomenon, or as a unilinear gradient. For the purpose of our discussion, at least three gradients need to be considered: (1) the orientation-disorientation quality, (2) wakefulness to sleep or coma quality, (3) judgment, evaluation and reflective self-awareness to hypersuggestibility, liability to wishful interpretation.

These qualities of consciousness can be influenced selectively by various drugs and other factors, and demonstrate a degree of independence. The differences in drugs in affecting these qualities often determine the choice of a drug.

ORIENTATION VERSUS DISORIENTATION

This dimension of awareness is most directly affected by the functional integrity of the brain. Under circumstances of disorientation a variety of affects may be displayed, often the expressive aspects of the affect alone, which, like "sham rage," would probably not have the ideational component or be the ordinary psychic event reflecting the meaning having an affect. On the other hand, the awareness of disorientation may generate either anxiety (and confusion) or exhilaration. Being freed from the task of orientation to reality is especially likely to be exhilarating when the disorientation is temporary and controlled, as in the "social" use of drugs. Disorientation may be used defensively as a block against confrontation or for carrying out a dangerous impulse. In functional amnesias, disorientation and dissociation become the major defenses (98). Drugs can be used for various kinds of dissociation, preventing either action or the recall and feeling of responsibility for action which has broken through. In either case, the dissociation occurs instead of anxiety or guilt. In modification of time-orientation, one can escape the urgency of unpleasant affects and the pressures of self-destructive or other threatening impulses. The modification of the body image permits the fantasy fulfillment of death, resurrection, and oceanic fusion yearnings. Ludwig and Levine have demonstrated in several studies that drugs, hypnosis, and psychotherapy can be used to modify these modalities, and thereby change the affective states (68 75).

Consciousness and the ego functions related to perception interpretation, hallucinatory and delusional experiences, are so subject to suggestion that it is often impossible to tell whether or not a pharmacological effect is involved. One such phenomenon is the "flashback" return of "LSD effects" weeks or months after its ingestion, and after returning to normal. The pharmacological mechanism by which LSD seems to manifest its function after its elimination from the brain is puzzling, and therefore insinuating that these late recurrences are also toxic. However, is it not just as likely that having experienced the fascinating and frightening alteration of consciousness induced by LSD, the same condition can become self-induced without the drug?

Petrie's experiments showed that the effects of alcohol and aspirin on sensory perceptions, including pain, were duplicated by placebo (94). Recently, studies of consciousness and its alteration by Silverman suggested that the aspects of attention which are subject to variation are (1) intensiveness or observed strength of stimuli, (2) extensiveness or scanning behavior, and (3) *selectiveness* field-dependency or the tendency to perceive in gestalt rather than detail. Silverman also pointed out that individuals in altered states of consciousness "perceive (minimal) stimuli stronger than normals do ('everything is much noisier and excites me'), but paradoxically minimize intense stimuli and are more tolerant of pain" (108). Thus sensory perception of high intensity or the intensification of perception of stimuli can be used to ward off painful affects, especially anxiety and depression, and thereby increase pain tolerance. Thus Silverman emphasizes the effects of modification of the perceptive and cognitive functions. Much experimental evidence shows the importance of these modifications in the defense against affects.

It has been demonstrated repeatedly that affects associated with a perception modify the reaction time and consciousness awareness of it. In tachistoscopic studies, subjects with experimentally induced medical anxiety (by receiving electric shock) responded with increased galvanic skin responses to the "previously shocked syllables over the indifferent ones even when exposure speeds were too rapid for conscious discrimination of the subject" (85). These authors have designated this type of subthreshold perceptional activity as "subception." McGinnies also showed in tachistoscopic studies that affect-laden words like "whore" or "penis" gave increasing galvanic responses, while the words tended to escape conscious recognition (86). Fisher has discussed the concept of perceptual defense, pointing out that reaction to a stimulus is on a preconscious level, associated with primary process cognition, and that affects may be produced even though the stimulus is not consciously recognized (33). In fact, patients selected for "high disturbance indicators (of aggression, homosexuality, and dependence) required longer exposure intervals for recognition of corresponding need-related TAT pictures than for mental pictures" (30).

In regard to attention, there are noted differences in function, and marked effects of drug use. Silverman states, "Field articulation responses of hypersensitive individuals, especially those in altered state of consciousness tend to be (a) global and diffuse rather than analytic, (b) strongly affected by minimal changes in internal and external stimuli stimulus conditions. In A. S. C. momentary fluctuations in attention are completely unpredictable . . . a sustained focus of attention . . . is impossible" (108). Dirkman has explained these phenomena as a "deautomatization of the psychological mechanisms which . . . organize, limit, select and interpret perceptual stimuli. Thinking is grossly subjective and egocentric; concepts are experienced as precepts. Causal relations may be perceived between most distantly related events, everything is capable of being connected with everything else in an irrational manner" (22).

The extensiveness of attention factor in altered states of consciousness shows a "preoccupation with a narrow circle of ideas . . . the range of environmental stimuli responded to is constricted markedly" (108). After a dose of 75 mgm of LSD, experimental subjects show a regression to infantile types of attention which are "object dominated"; there is "minimal scanning behavior," lack of interest in distant "background," and "overvaluation of close dominant stimulus" (108). This is in contrast to the "centration effect" of normal adults, who compensate by scanning the distant field and psychologically overestimate the distant background data (39). In general, under the influence of drugs such as LSD, or in trauma states, "individuals who are hypersensitive to minimum stimulation 'require' a compensatory adjustment (under-responsiveness) to protect themselves from strong stimulation" (52). The result is that the hyperattention to the minimal stimuli acts as a distraction and protection against painful affects and threatening ideas.

An example of how this is accomplished has been found in changes in the saccadic eye movements. These rapid flick-like jumps of the eye occur on the average of once or twice per second during fixation on a given field; in states of concentration, they are essential for detail vision. However, in altered states of consciousness, there is an increase of saccadic eye movement, with a redundancy of detail information sampling and over-estimation of irrelevant detail, at the expense of concentration at the relevant perception. Silverman points out that these changes in the perceptual function may account for the reports of increased clarity of vision but at the same time in the restruction of the field and its relevance (108).

Thus the somatic perceptual apparatus may be modified in its function, resulting in a variety of ways in which the orientation and the meaning of the situation may be changed. Nor do these phenomena occur only under the influence of drugs, they are in fact part of those functions which can heighten the stimulus barrier, and may take place under a variety of conditions. Shor has reported that in a study of a "normal college population," he found most subjects to have experienced spontaneously and "naturally" a variety of "hypnotical phenomena" consisting of a "relative suspension of reality orientation" (107).

That one is able to modify one's perception should not surprise us. Indeed, the emphatic denial of this ability is of theoretical interest, because it represents a need to deny that our cognitive and perceptive processes are influenced by emotions and repressed conflictual material. The liberal arts students described by Shor had a lesser need to deny and/or control the occurrence of lapses of control of their consciousness than engineering students, because they were presumably freer to use their imagination and to be more introspective (107). In fact, most of the signs and symptoms were those we classify as mental illness. From that point of view, it might be said that to maintain one's sanity is equivalent with the need to protect the integrity of one's consciousness and related ego function. Indeed, many people live in dread of such disturbances and a survey of "acute psychoses" revealed many "psychedelic experiences" as reported by the patients of Bowers and Freedman. These authors adduced the common experience in both acute psychoses and psychedelic experiences to be "heightened consciousness or awareness." They describe the patients during the nascent stages of their reported psychosis as having "stepped beyond the restrictions of the usual awareness," but at the same time being frightened by the experience (13).

The impending psychosis can be considered in terms of a breakthrough of hitherto repressed impulses, which as a last resort are warded off by the "false insight." Since this effect is facilitated by drugs, after its discovery upon drug use, it may become more accessible and utilizable simply because the dread of becoming overwhelmed with the "breakthrough" is lessened. From the point of view of cathectic energy, in acute psychosis, dreams, and drug use there is a shift of cathexes from the "outside" to the body sensory apparatus and its mental representation and preconscious mode of cognition. This shift may become so gratifying under the pressure of emotional conflicts that its recurrence is yearned for.

In their study of the effect of alcohol intake on alcoholics as compared to depressives and controls, Mayfield and Allen stated that the alcoholics did not report a subjective relief from depression, but showed "deterioration," notably disorientation (78). They interpreted their findings as casting doubt on the idea that alcoholics were obtaining relief from depression or anxiety by drinking. However, it would appear to us more likely that in the alcoholics they studied there was a greater utilization of disorientation for relief from unpleasant affect. This becomes even more apparent in the use of psychedelic drugs for the purpose of escaping unpleasant states, because the major effect of these drugs is in blocking normal orientation and encouraging hallucinatory experiences.

WAKEFULNESS TO SLEEP STATES SPECTRUM

The idea of total anesthesia into the oblivion of sleep applies to the relief of painful affects, just as it does to surgical operations or physical pain. In fact, somnolence is sought relatively rarely, and then usually for the enjoyment of dream states. However, when wakefulness is not considered as an all-or-none phenomenon but as a gradient of states, the hypnotic manner of relief from unpleasant states becomes more apparent. It is a commonplace observation among drug abusers, including alcoholics, that the persons who are driven to reach oblivion as fast as possible were subject to a malignant course in their drug dependence. The

"nods" of the heroin user is an instance of intensive anesthesia, and incidentally, also of the libidination of the
moment and sensation of falling asleep. The close connec-
tions between the mechanism of wakefulness, arousal, and
anxiety may offer much fruitful information. It is possible
that with some drugs, such as alcohol, the inhibition of full
wakefulness and alertness is a potent means of blocking the
affect of anxiety. On the other hand, when drugs such as
the amphetamines are used, they produce both a super-
wakefulness and a state of physiological anxiety which are
utilized in a manic-type defense against depression.

Perhaps the question of whether manic or somnolent defenses against anxious-depression, or more accurately the
precursor of these affects, are preferred depends on the
person's ability to deal with the ideation related to the
affect. If the painful ideas can be reversed, denied, or re-
placed with other interests, a manic defense is possible. If
not, the stimulated depressed patient may develop agitated
depression or be driven to suicide. The psycho-motor re-
tardation is a defense against such action. The relief sought
here is sleep. However, the inability to turn one's mind to
hypocathected (indifferent) ideas precludes natural falling
off to sleep. A commonly seen interference is the presence
of physical pain, even of very low intensity, or dysphoric
affect with obsessions.

The function of wakefulness is also related to the energy
available for dealing with the intrapsychic and external
reality. Cathectic energy is necessary for conscious perceptions and the formation of memory traces; a higher level of
cathexis for a conscious memory (90 98). Adequate
cathexis of this function is required to make a mental event
conscious cognition, otherwise there is a dream or night-

mare-like phenomenon. In regard to drug abusers, there is a selectively high cathexis of the mental apparatus related to the sensory functions, as part of the general fixation on the elusive "outside" object and the source of supplies. Under these circumstances it becomes especially urgent to block the function of consciousness, and with it the impact of reflective self-awareness. To put it another way, because of the yearning for finding and introjecting the object-representation which has remained external, the sensory perceptions create a "hunger" for supplies which becomes unbearable. The dilemma is to create a state in which one is alert to the pleasurable perceptions but not the unpleasant ones—to perceive only pleasurable inner states but to block the unpleasant one. However, as the life-style of the drug dependent person diminishes the opportunities of gratification and enjoyment from without, and pleasant affects from within, there is a gradual shift to sacrificing his alertness and ability for enjoyment or the prize of blocking the un-pleasure. The infantile goals of the oral stage—as summarized in Lewin's triad: to eat, to be eaten, and to go off to sleep—become predominant (70). The wish for total relief of tension and sleep is most conspicuous.

SELF-AWARENESS

Since we are concerned with those aspects of consciousness related to affects, we wish to stress reflective self-awareness, and those aspects of self-perception by which the meaning of affect can become conscious and verbalized. We have discussed above the advantages of verbalization of affect as a protection against somatic stress. In addition, however, when the meaning of the affect and of the conflict behind it is not consciously known, one has to make up an explanation as to its cause and meaning. For instance, anxiety equivalents are sometimes experienced as a "heart attack," the danger being death, and the cause attributed to whatever current unconscious fantasies dictate (66). If the somatic components of affects can be experienced without such portent, they may be accepted as "thrills," as we mentioned in Chapter I.

The use of drugs modifies the experience by the combination of physiological and psychological effects. Reflective self-awareness—orientation and recognition of actual intrapsychic tension—is suppressed. At the same time, the usual inhibitions against out-and-out wish fullfillment fantasy are blocked. Certain types of fantasies are made possible by taking the drug which symbolizes the fusion between the "good" self-representation and the idealized object-representation. This set of circumstances gives one such a feeling of invulnerability that the physiological components of anxiety can be experienced with pleasure, and without threat. This is more obvious in the use of Khat or amphetamine, which produces norepinephrine release or effect, but is also quite clearly observable with the use of Cannabis.

Our previous reasoning in regard to the importance of anxiety and the perception of danger in regard to pain tolerance is confirmed by the work of Kurland and co-workers in demonstrating that with the use of LSD, analgesic and the blocking of the fear of dying were achieved in terminal cancer patients (67). Thus, not only in neurotic anxiety, but in the very approach of death, the impact of the affect can be modified by the blocking or modification of the *meaning* of the event or perception. Religious ecstasy as a bulwark against pain shows that such modifications can be achieved without drugs, by suggestion or persuasion. Moslems are alleged to have gone to their death in holy wars joyously because it promised eternal libidinal gratification. This is an example of the modification of the interpretation of a situation (by denial and flight into fantasy), thereby substituting joyous for anxious expectations.

Modification of superego function

However, the expression of affects under the influence of drugs has some "phony," some "incomplete" nature, as is best illustrated by the "crying in one's beer" mechanism. Under those circumstances, the unpleasant affect is not blocked, not changed, but the ego is modified so as to permit affective expression. This is accomplished by displacing the ideational components to trivial ones. The original conflicts thus remain isolated, and the affect will continue to be generated. However, the gain in blocking self-awareness is in the ego ideal. Often "having feelings" is experienced as a threat to one's adult, especially masculine, identity. Thus the shame of crying or sentimentality can be blocked. However, the most difficult problem is that when potential affects are of a primitive type, predominantly somatic affect precursors, the threat of becoming overwhelmed with them is greater than when dealing with matured, verbalized desomatized affects. Because these affects are so rigidly warded off, they are experienced as "attacks" of destructive potential. In chronic depressive problems the punitive and destructive meaning can thus be reinterpreted.

Note the following self-observation by the nineteenth-century poet-hashish-taker Baudelaire. He describes how a hashish taker, reveling in feelings of "superiority to all mankind," suddenly recalls a guilt and shame-ridden memory:

> But you can be sure that the hashish here will courageously confront these reproachful phantoms. He will even know how to extract new elements of pleasure and of pride from these hideous memories. His rationalization will go something like this: once the first sensation of pain is gone, he will analyze with curiosity the remembered deed or the feeling that is troubling his present glory. He will study the motivation of that past action, the circumstances that surrounded him. If he doesn't find in these circumstances sufficient reasons to absolve him or at least to minimize his sin, don't let yourself imagine that he feels defeated! I can watch his reasoning as if it were a mechanical device under a transparent glass: "This ridiculous deed, cowardly or vile, whose memory has troubled me a moment, is in complete contradiction with my true self, my present self, and the energy even I show in condemning it, the inquisitorial care I take in analyzing and judging it prove my noble and divine aptitudes for virtue. How many men do you think you can find who are this skillful in self-judgment, this severe in self-condemnation?" Not only does he condemn himself, but he glorifies himself . . . He completely mixes up dream and deed. His imagination gets more and more excited before this enchanting spectacle of his own self, improved and idealized. He substitutes this fascinating illusion of himself for his real self that is so poor in willpower, so rich in vanity. He finally decrees his own deification in clear and simple terms. Before him he sees a world of abominable joys: "I am the most virtuous of men!" (5)

One of the most complex functions involved in affect is that of memory. In problems of chronic depression, anxiety or boredom, the underlying conflicts represent memories in the broader sense, including unconscious memory traces. The blocking of memories would be one way to prevent the development of affects.* Drive derivatives require association with memory traces in order to reach a level of cathexis and elaboration to achieve consciousness. The most common instance of such a use of tranquilizers is to block obsessions and delusions, dreams and recollections, or to reduce the level of mental energy available (93).

However, the translation of concepts from the pharmacological to the psychological poses the danger of such confusion that we must handle this proposition very carefully. One of the problems introduced here is that the very same drugs which might lower the energic level of the ego might also lower the intensity of the countercathexes and signal anxiety, and therefore make possible the emergence of memories of impulses. Our experience shows that the effect produced depends not only on the choice of the drug but also upon the personality of the user. There is a consistent pattern in drug users, such as in alcoholics, so that some drink themselves into oblivion, whereas others indulge in either affect-free or drug numbed "pseudo-affect," such as "crying in one's beer." Still others achieve a temporary suspension of superego function which, coupled with a corruption of the superego by later punishment, permits the acting out of a variety of impulses.

The suspension of the superego function achieved by the drug acts not only in the prohibitive and punitive

* After all, the great contribution of Freud in *Inhibition, Symptoms and Anxiety* is to show that repression is accomplished within the ego upon the perception of signal anxiety, and in order to prevent the danger of traumatization (38).

functions, but on the ego-ideal as well, and the function of the evaluation of the meaning of any act, mediated through the ego, results in changes in the usual inter-systemic regulatory functions.

Case illustration

> A patient wondered why he kept taking heroin. He related that he tried to "stay off the stuff" for two weeks after his last discharge, but he started feeling "loose and scared." During the last month he began to feel as if people were talking about him and pointing at him. At times he felt "like there is something crawling around in my head." There were also frequent auditory hallucinations, especially during the week prior to admission. For example: "You are a dope fiend . . . you black SOB." However, when he is "high" these do not bother him. He states that he just ignores them.

We have mentioned that one of the effects of the changed state of consciousness is the change of the body image. The most direct way to change the body image and ego is to change the condition of the body, as in anesthetization, as seen by the following example:

> A man who had used the drug to ward off his passive yearnings, and to overcompensate his masculine function, also used the drug (Demerol) to extend his ability to carry on intercourse, and to perform work to athletic proportions. The fact of his "Superman" activity was then utilized to ward off the anxiety over his passive yearnings and latent anxiety about his masculine function.

In the drugs which produce perceptual distortions, a significant wishfulfillment consists in the modification of body image. This function is especially gratifying in the presence of anxiety about one's acceptability, especially in adolescence. However, it is also manifest in other ways. For instance, the claim of the tremendous sexual potency with the use of LSD, as in the case where the ingestant was actually found to have spent the "trip" cowering in a corner. It is this mechanism which may result in the feeling of "liberation" from one's body and transcendental fusion with the spiritual world.

Modification of body image and body function

In general, drug dependent persons tend toward a hyper-cathexis of the perceptive system, a dominance by it in their orientation. Their way of dealing with problems could be conceptualized as their manipulating their sensory, perceptive, and interpretive functions, instead of dealing with the real sources of their unpleasant affects by problem resolution or adaptive changes. Knapp has pointed out that sensory perception in dreams substitute and defend against certain affects (57). Psychoanalysts in general are familiar with the very brightly colored dream representing a defense against depression in its latent content, or a humorous dream as a defense against aggression. Murphy extended this point, showing that certain sensory perceptions may represent the pregenital defenses against genitality, and that fixation on traumata related to specific sensory perceptions makes the development of a mature genital character impossible. He states that "all activities involving sensory organs have their narcissistic and ego-defensive aspects" (83).

Indeed, we pointed out in Chapter II that the insistence on the identity of the drug with the object is a major unconscious basis of the problems of drug dependence. We also pointed out the drug user's insistence that "his world," as he experiences it under the influence of drugs, is superior to the "real" or "square" world and is *in fact* the ultimate reality. This reaction is not the basic misinterpretation of the state of affairs. The basic "delusion" is the insistence on the identity of the perception with the object.

In comparing a drug dependent person to a neurotic, we find that both suffer an introversion and fixation on an incestuous love object. However, they differ in that the neurotic hypercathects his memories and fantasies, whereas the person given to drug abuse hypercathects the perceptory system. In fact, the drug user seems to have a fear of ideas and words, and seeks a regression to pre-verbal, hallucinatory experiences, such as visual, auditory, or tactile ones. The enchantment with the psychedelic perceptual distortions is not only with their unusual nature, but with the pre-verbal affect and self-representation modification. One is reminded of the reaction of the schizophrenic person in reacting to words as being identical with the object and dread of destruction, regressing to pre-verbal cognition as well.

The drug user produces within himself a condition similar to a psychosis or to a dream state, but his basic motivation is different. The schizophrenic, caught up in terrifying fantasies that threaten to destroy himself and his world, regresses to the world of fantasy in order to render himself helpless and thus avert the danger. He is not primarily interested in the modification of his consciousness or orientation (a fact which we use for the differential diagnosis between functional and organic psychosis), but his relationship with his reality. However, the drug user is interested in the modification of his *consciousness primarily as a method of modifying his affective states.*

SUMMARY

In the pursuit of modifying the emotional state and avoidance of painful affect, one can take advantage of a variety of drug effects, and achieve the final result through a variety of methods. Among these possibilities some common patterns can be evolved.

(1) Anesthesia and analgesia, in which the pain of the affect, its physiological aspect, is blocked, as in the use of narcotics. This is basically a hypnotic method, in the sense that consciousness is reduced till the extreme case in which sleep is produced. As wakefulness is sacrificed, the ideational components of affects are at first reduced to dreams, and then abolished. The blocking of both the superego and the awareness of the intersystemic tension is probably the most common relief sought.

(2) Reinterpretation of the psychic conflict, or change of the self-image. By the use of drugs which suppress critical cognition and disturb perception, it is possible to reinterpret one's psychic reality so as to ameliorate, change, or reverse one's affect into its opposite. This type of reaction is especially common in the use of psychedelic drugs, and has been used by man for ages in religious, mystical, and other ecstasies. The basic modification is in the ideas of self, the world, the meaning of one's state. This can be observed in the claim that certain drugs are "mind expanding" to deny the need to suppress or distort the painful self-awareness.

(3) Disorientation and dissociation. Among the number of ego functions involved in the conscious aspects of affect production, the function of reality testing, and reflective self-awareness, the drug use is directed to some degree of confusion or dissociation. The temporary relinquishing of the task of orientation is experienced as a relief. Beyond this, in some drug dependent personalities the dissociations permit the avoidance of anxiety over action or impulses, which are handled by "splitting off" and repression.

(4) Modification of physical function—usually applicable where certain functions, such as excessive work or sexual activity, are used to ward off unacceptable passive yearnings. The primary "addiction" is to work, or to phallic overcompensation which has to be bolstered up chemically. A variation of this is the use of drugs to relieve muscle or other aches produced by the work or tension, or to achieve some pleasant physical sensation in individuals who had to cut themselves off from most pleasures and gratifications.

IV
implications for therapy

Our study of selected aspects of the problems of drug dependence obviously does not make possible a comprehensive picture of the therapy in the entire field. However, there are some implications upon therapy that need to be considered. In fact, we have been unable to resist digressing into discussing some therapeutic aspects along the way. For instance, we pointed out that the extreme ambivalence, and specifically the dread of aggressive wishes, may make the dyadic situation unbearable. For that reason some types of drug dependent persons may require treatment in a clinic, or group therapy at least, in the beginning. We referred to previous work by Krystal and associates in which the necessity and utility of probation as a backdrop to treatment were explored (62). This technique is related to the drug dependent patient's need to "wall off" and externalize his superego, and the relationship between the ego and its object- and self-representations.

As usual, the theories presented were the product of psychotherapy with drug dependent patients and serve to explain the phenomena we observed during treatment. The following is a case illustration of such an event:

> A patient dependent upon the use of narcotics related that
> during his first attempt of psychotherapy several years previ-

ously, he was given an interpretation to the effect that he yearned to be passively gratified by a man. Although his passive yearnings were interpreted in connection with a dream which made these needs fairly explicit, the patient responded with intense anxiety mounting to a panic state. In the subsequent days and years this fear of the return of the intense anxiety was a major cause for his increasing his use of the narcotics, as well as self-destructive behavior which destroyed his marriage and greatly damaged his business.

Although his treatment with the first psychiatrist continued for several months after the above interpretation, the rising tide of anxiety could not be stemmed. The patient's condition became so severe that he had to be hospitalized for a long time. Fairly soon after release he relapsed into the use of the drug. When he finally reentered psychotherapy, it was necessary to deal with disturbances in ego functions especially related to his ability to deal with anxiety and the affect precursors of a more primitive nature.

In the beginning of the treatment after his discharge from the hospital, he was able to maintain business pressures at a lower level, and got by without any drug or medication. However, as the pressures of his work, family, and treatment mounted, he started to use alcohol in a pattern reproducing his use of narcotics. Since he was able to keep it within manageable limits, the use of the alcohol was tolerated. Although the use of Antabuse to block the alcohol intake was considered, the therapist (Krystal) decided against it, feeling that it was best to avoid an accumulation of affect to the point were the patient might feel threatened with being overwhelmed again. More importantly, however, the patient's use and struggle with the alcohol in an intermediate stage of the transference made possible the observation and interpretation of the uses and meaning of the drug to him. In his first psychotherapeutic experience he was able to experience those feelings in the transference to the therapist.

We shall not go into the details of the question of requirements of abstinence in the treatment of patients in whom drug use is a problem. Krystal has dealt with it else-where, reviewing what factors need to be considered in making an individual evaluation in this respect (60). Neither will we concern ourselves with the dynamics of the homosexual panic which developed. In patients of this type a long preparatory period may be necessary before threatening material, or material which brings on a great quantity of painful affect, can be dealt with. The period of preliminary work is designed to let the patient become aware of his fear of these feelings, and the fact that they are self-limiting, non-destructive, but part of the normal function—as a patient said of his anxiety, "like racing my engine." Thus, gradually the pain tolerance is increased primarily in regard to affects, but to other painful experiences as well, especially frustrations.

A PREPARATORY PHASE OF TREATMENT SERVING TO INCREASE AFFECT TOLERANCE

Needless to say, the interpretation given to the above patient should have been "from the ego side," alerting him to his fears of certain impulses. The rules of good therapy are certainly applicable here. But the issue is that by precept the therapist thus teaches the patient to approach his impulses and feelings gradually, to aim for and practice the mastery of his affects and needs. Affects are primarily drive derivatives, and they also represent an instinctual need for expression. It follows that the very same goal and technique which we have recommended for helping the patient deal with his affects also apply to his difficulties with instinct gratification. We have pointed out that the disturbance in this sphere is a major cause of drug dependence. The success in the patient's dealing with his feelings makes him more capable of instinctual gratification.

In making judgments about the nature of modifications and/or parameters necessary to make possible the continuation of the therapy, the ego functions described above are an addition to the consideration one exercises in the treatment of neurotic patients. A preliminary or preparatory phase of treatment is necessary in all but the primarily neurotic drug users. It is impossible to totally avoid dealing with emerging material, but it may have to be "interpreted upward," with some temporizing, to allow the patient to build up the related ego functions. This procedure is analogous to the treatment of the "borderline" or psychotic patient, but preparation is concerned with somewhat different issues and ego functions. During this phase the therapist serves the double role of discovering the nature of the patient's ego disturbances, and of helping him to deal with affects, sometimes by explanations and instructions. For instance, in relationship to anxiety it is necessary to demonstrate to the patient its nature as a feeling and how his fear of it perpetuates and multiplies it. This and other reactions to "having" affects have been discussed above for the purpose of providing tools in increasing the patient's tolerance of painful affects.

During this phase of the treatment considerable activity and interference in the patient's life may be necessary, in some cases in order to bring down the level of painful Ur-affects to the point where the patient can learn to tolerate them without drugs. For instance, modifications in the patient's work, social, or marital relations may be suggested or even instituted by the therapist. The principle of non-communication with relatives cannot be observed because of the above, and because they must feel free to inform the therapist of the patient's relapses or acute emergencies. If these modifications become so severe that it is felt that "too much has happened" in actually forcing the therapist into a parental role to make possible later the analysis of the transference, then a change of therapists (preferably to another member of the clinic) can and should be made, after careful preparation and after the reaction to loss and rejection is worked out with the original therapist.

While in the preliminary, preparatory phase, the treatment can be described as supportive and didactic in part. It is not supportive at all if the therapist fails to interpret and deal with those impulses which have broken through into the preconscious part of the ego, particularly those which have been acted out. Failure to do so not only deprives the patient of the opportunity to attempt conscious mastery of his impulses (especially aggression), but also gives him the terrifying feeling that his therapist, too, is afraid of his aggression and is willing to enter a conspiracy of silence about it. Moreover, Krystal has pointed out in the past that counter-transference problems tend to make physicians treating drug withdrawal states reenact the behavior of the patient's mother; not to attend to his *specific needs* but either angrily reject him, ignore him, or overtreat him with sedative drugs (59). The same transference and counter-transference reactions take place in psychotherapy, and may be acted out in giving unnecessary support or insisting on the total discontinuation of the use of the drug (60).

THE PROHIBITION BY COMMAND AND PHARMACOLOGICAL AGENTS

One special technique used in the treatment of drug dependent persons contains elements of probation (i. e., adding "external" controls) and enforces abstinence. By giving Antabuse or similarly acting medication to the alcoholic, or by conditioning the patient to react adversely to any drug, the situation is produced whereby upon taking the drug the patient develops a sort of poisoning. What we have discussed so far necessitates that we consider two meanings of the effect on the patient:

(1) The sudden deprivation of the relief and support from the drug confronts the patient with the dreaded painful affect in a massive dose. Rado has pointed out that where this occurs, when the drug loses its effectiveness it creates a panic within the patient which he has called the "pharmacothymic crisis" (95). This situation revives some of the most profound fears of the patient—notably, being abandoned and helpless. Krystal pointed out that the rage involved leads to either destructive acting out or panic (including psychosis such as alcoholic hallucinosis), and that it produces a severe physiological stress reaction (59 61 63). Hence, the careful evaluation of the patient's ego function is necessary before such a step is undertaken. Modifications of the procedure (e.g., gradual withdrawal from the drug; temporary substitutions of relieving but less euphoriant drugs) can be used, but it is necessary that during this time the patient be prepared for giving up of the drug, and his ego functions related to painful affects tolerance be improved.

(2) In making the drug capable of producing severe symptoms, and incapable of giving relief, we are in fact making real one of the most profound fears of the drug dependent person. We have discussed in detail the nature of the ambivalence to the drug as an object-representation substitute, and the guilt and fear associated with taking it. To render the drug poisonous is so close to the patient's conflict and fears on the cannibalistic level of his oral fantasies that it may be terrifying to him. This act must be experienced as outright sadism on the part of the therapist. This type of reaction by the patient used to be further confirmed when doctors insisted on giving alcoholics a "test dose" of alcohol after Antabuse. If the drug is experienced as a substitute for the maternal, sustaining object-representation, the therapist, as its poisoner and depriver of the patient's ability to get relief, must deal with such reactions and fantasies in the transference. The loss of the object substitute in a forcible fashion, whether by the use of drugs or suggestion, creates a situation ripe for suicide. Just when he is "doing great" the patient may give vent to his aggression and yearning to be reassured of love by a suicide attempt.

THE PROBLEM OF COUNTER-TRANSFERENCE

With these patients the problems of counter-transference are especially difficult because of the aggression they include (82 106). Because patients are very demanding, expressing insatiable, "endless" oral fantasies, the analyst has to deal with their fears of being devoured or destroyed, and often becomes overly concerned with "giving" too much or too little to them. These reactions must be identified and dealt with by the therapist lest they prevent him from recognizing the patients' specific needs and conflicts, and from supplying the explanations that may improve the ego-functions related to dealing with the painful affects in their regressed form.

FACILITATING THE ESTABLISHMENT OF A BENIGN INTROJECT

The importance of regression in regard to affects cannot be overstressed. The causes and results of dedifferentiation, resomatization and primitivization of the underlying fantasies, become an important objective of the psychotherapeutic work. The regression to magical thinking perpetuates the dread of one's aggression and the need to perpetuate the rigid encapsulation of the object-representation. The following case illustrates the point:

> A patient, now in his second analysis, kept reporting verbatim what his first analyst had said, "in quotation marks" as it were, without having utilized or assimilated anything the first analyst said. Often he made demands for something to be said to him, but forever remained "hungry," being unable to "digest" or use anything he was told. It became apparent that to do so would mean the destruction of the object, and the result would be his own death as a "motherless child." He constantly warded off impulses to destroy the analyst and take away all his power and love, but because of his dread of his impulses, he also felt it a necessity for his survival to preserve the analyst as somebody "out there" who loved him and thereby granted him permission to live, eat, and enjoy life. In the following dream he illustrated this conflict. "I was in my boss's house, arguing with him. Everybody was going into

the other room to eat, but I was standing there, not knowing if it was all right for me to go to eat."

His association started with a long list of grievances against his boss, but led to his recognition that he wanted the boss's house, wife, shop, money, power—"everything." As he talked about this feeling, he protested that these wishes were not from greed but "hunger" and he felt his mouth as he spoke. The feeling of deprivation, that eating and other gratifications were prohibited to him, referred to the specific time in his life when his family fell apart as a result of his mother's mental illness, and he was terribly deprived.

Another part of the dream dealt with his fantasies of having caused it all by his destructive impulses. In fact, the particular dream referred to attacking the mother's "insides" with his penis and teeth, and destroying them with his excreta, the destruction including his yet unborn younger sister.

He never could develop any comfort or confidence that his aggression was controllable or safely manageable by him, because as a child he blamed himself for destroying his mother and the family. Subsequently, he stayed in many homes, and each time he had to be moved he felt he had "eaten" himself out of "family and home" again, and had destroyed these parents too. He was so severely traumatized that he has lived in dread of the return of the trauma. The dread was experienced in various terms, as in the dream that his aggression would make the boss hate him and throw him out. Under these circumstances, since no living objects could be trusted, only "things," especially drugs, became reliable sources of succor, and being inanimate, they were safe from his aggression. He was especially habituated to the use of a fairly large amount of hypnotics. He knew the exact moment when the drug took effect, when he'd sigh deeply, and then he'd have pleasurable "goose flesh" and other anxiety equivalent sensations. He would then enjoy the increasing drowsiness, all of which served as a sort of decrescendo foreplay to falling asleep, even prolonging it by fighting sleep. Finally, feeling satiated, he'd fall asleep. The ingestion of the drug object-substitute gave him the feeling of satiation, drowsiness, and permitted sleep. However, as he experienced the drug as a transubstantiation of the object, he felt very guilty about taking it and fearful that it would harm him, and he experienced this fear each time immediately upon feeling the drug taking effect. This reaction expressed the wish to be eaten by the object, thus completing the oral triad described by Lewin (70).

In his relationship with the first therapist, the patient could not use the therapist's interpretations or their content and meaning because his destructive impulses were not dealt with in the transference. The affect disturbances also escaped recognition and verbalization *because* they were in the form of the Ur-affect, the primary affect of displeasure. However, he was able to use the therapist's speaking to him as feeding, and therefore love, a permission to do and enjoy things. As a result, he advanced his career and other aspects of his life at that time.

This patient's use of the transference, not for work in the therapy but to manage his life more comfortably, is a manifestation of what Fenichel called the "object-addiction" (32). Drug dependent patients may, without formal treatment, arrive at a point when they are able to use a person, a situation, even an ideology—some "external"—to create an object-representation which they can utilize for inspiration and achieving a major change in their identity and function. These events of conversion are analogous to various religious experiences and the "existential crisis" (77). In such events occurring in groups dedicated to "fighting the devil-drug," there may occur a rupture of the encapsulation of the object-representation, and a patient now identified with the depriving mother, may be driven to spend all his energy depriving other people of the drug and denouncing the former substitute for the love object (drug) with the reproaches which are applicable to the love object of his infancy and childhood.

SOLO THERAPY VERSUS TREATMENT IN A CLINIC

As we have pointed out before, the problem of object loss has to be considered with special care in these cases. It poses, for instance, a serious obstacle to the success of psychotherapy in clinics in which the staff keeps changing. All too often the patient also drops out after his therapist leaves. Where this is anticipated, an auxilliary therapist should be introduced early, and a secondary relationship can be established according to his discipline (e.g., periodic psychological testing), just to maintain the "spare" relationship. The death of a close relative is a major psychological crisis, at which time a relapse of some kind can be expected.

The problem of object-loss is most persistent and troublesome in youth. Anny Katan has most precisely described that in adolescence, in contrast to displacement of the incestuous tie to the parent, the "removal" defined as "abolishing incestuous ties once and for all" is the process which makes possible the freedom to love, and maturation into adult roles (53). This removal is accomplished by work analogous to mourning, and is experienced as a painful loss. This pain of adolescence is the very reason why the young are so tempted to use drugs, and simultaneously the very reason why they cannot afford to do it without interfering with their accomplishment of the adolescent work of mourning and removal. In this regard, again the problem is related to the imperfect development of their ego function, especially in regard to the development of tolerance of unpleasant states such as pain, painful affect, tension, and the frustrations of work. Thus the anhedonic uses of drugs in adolescence represent a challenge to our ability to prepare patients for confrontations and struggles with their own emotions.

AGGRESSION IN DRUG DEPENDENT INDIVIDUALS

In general, considering the use of drugs for the relief of painful affects and states necessitates a reconsideration of the framework of therapy. There are three separate concepts involved: drug use, drug abuse, and drug dependence. In and of itself drug dependence is an inconvenience, as it limits the patient's freedom and self-reliance. However, in and of itself it does not become a major problem except where coupled with the phenomenon of tolerance for more drugs, with an increased preoccupation with obtaining it, causing changes in the patient's life-style and goals. What we observe under these circumstances is a *failure* of the drug to maintain a comfortable and workable adjustment. Krystal has pointed out that the successful drug user is able to handle the problems of drug tolerance by periodic withdrawal, and experiencing during the withdrawal period the otherwise suppressed physiological aspects of the affects (63). Thus, the drug users who come to our attention are those who are unsuccessful at it.

There are some drug users who have a malignant course

apparently "from the beginning," and this is both in their rapid increase in quantity of drugs used, total absorption with the drug, rapid deterioration of all object-representation ties, not eating, and often frequent involvement in physical injury as a result of fights or "accidents." However, for the most part, even in such cases, one can find a point in which the nature of the drug user takes a malignant turn. We do not disagree with Karl Menninger's point of view that some addictions are a matter of chronic suicide (80).

What we have been discussing in terms of affect tolerance was by definition about the handling of instinct derivatives, the dealing with aggression, self-destructive impulses and the fear of them, which is subject to the vicissitudes we have mentioned. While the feeling of anger is one of these painful affects, the tolerance of which is impaired in drug dependent people, there are specific problems of dealing with aggression because of the magical thinking which we discussed in connection *with* the self- and object-representation. The following case illustrates this type of difficulty:

> From childhood on the patient had a family and environmental history in which violence played a part. At home, physical abuse was the method of discipline; in the neighborhood, it took him till his adolescence before he was able to fight off the bullies and assure his safety. He was a football player with a history of serious injuries.
>
> His first marriage was a frustrating one, both sexually and affectively. When he discovered that his wife was an alcoholic, he himself took to drugs and a variety of activities which virtually destroyed his career. While most of the time he would take abuse in silence, on occasion he would become violent to the point that only luck prevented him from homicide.

His second marriage evolved a similar pattern. His wife would heap abuse upon him, which he took in silence, bolstered by the use of drugs. Whenever he felt assaulted, he'd take the drug with a self-destructive, revengeful, but also anger-suppressing intent. It became clear that his inability to defend himself was significantly related to his fear that if he relinquished his self-control, and total suppression of angry reactions, he might become overwhelmed with his anger and kill his wife. In fact, the couple engaged in a sort of Russian roulette in which periodically the outbreak of aggression threatened their survival in a variety of ways.

Most drug users get along well for a long time with their drug dependence, and use the drug to support their function. For those who end up in the psychiatrist's office, there has been a turning point in which the drug can no longer be handled to deal with their problems, and the "complications" of drug use become rapidly conspicuous. It is, therefore, essential that in evaluating a drug user for psychotherapy, we discover not only what he uses the drug for, but also if his using it creates problems, and what are the causes of the failure of the drug.

As mentioned above, the loss of a love-object-representation, real, symbolic, or by change of relation, may be an event which triggers the deterioration. However, we must add to this previously described problem our theories about the drug user as a traumatized individual whose dread of the return of the traumatization makes him very susceptible to a variety of difficulties. Such individuals are quite masochistic, and if things go well for them, they may develop increasing anxiety. They tend to link any misfortunes in their lives together, attributing to them the meaning, "the day of judgment has arrived." Indeed, the unconscious fantasy precipitating the change in one's ability to support one's function with the use of a drug is so complex and varied that an individual determination of it is essential. The change in the course of drug dependence is indeed an emergency in the sense that a hitherto repressed fantasy, conflict or danger *emerges,* and it behooves us to discover it and deal with it.

Even the apparently simple cause-and-effect matters of drug use should not be presumed "typical." For instance, we cannot take it for granted that because of the use of Cannabis, the "Heads" lose their ambition. Perhaps the drug was taken in the first place because of anxiety encountered when they were trying to advance themselves, and the drug—allowing a revision of their goals—simply permits them to convert the anxiety into an inhibition. But, behind the inhibition there are varied fantasies, conflicts, and character traits of the person. We do feel that one should suspect and look for a history of early traumatization, which greatly intensifies anxiety and makes the possibility of disaster more credible. The traumatization also impairs ego functions related to dealing with anxiety, so that these individuals do worse rather than better when under pressure. Last but not least, the traumatization represents a narcissistic injury which seriously impaired their self-confidence.

Far more important, however, is the problem we discussed in Chapter II, namely, that the quest for the symbolic reunion with the alienated love-object-representation is doomed to failure and repetition. Still, we must bear in mind that many people manage to keep this yearning in check for long periods of time by ingestion or injection of one drug or another, and that those who come to our attention are the people for whom this self-maintaining operation has failed. Therefore, understanding the causes and meanings of that failure should be an early quest in psychotherapy.

references

(1) Abelson, R., A. Ginsberg, and M. Wyshograd, "Psychedelics and Religion: a Symposium." *Humanist,* pp. 153–56, Sept.–Dec. 1967.

(2) Archibald, H. E., *et al.,* "Gross Stress Reaction in Combat, a Fifteen Year Follow-Up." *Am. J. Psych.* 119: 317–21, 1962.

(3) Arlow, J., and R. Brenner, *Psychoanalytic Concepts and the Structural Theory.* N.Y., Int. U. Press, 1964.

(4) Bak, R. C., "Schizophrenic Defense Against Aggression." *Int. J. Psychoan.* 35: 1–6, 1959.

(5) Baudelaire, C., quoted by C. B. Osborn, "Artificial Paradises: Baudelaire and the Psychedelic Experience." *Am. Scholar* 37: 660–68, 1968.

(6) Beecher, H. K., "The Powerful Placebo." *J.A.M.A.* 159: 1602–05, 1955.

(7) —— "Evidence for Increased Effectiveness of Placebo with Increased Stress." *Am. J. Phys.* 187: 163–69, 1956.

(8) —— "The Relationship of Wounds to Pain Experienced." *J.A.M.A.* 197: 1609–13, 1956.

(9) —— "The Subjective Response and Reaction to Sensation." *Am. J. Med.* 20: 107–13, 1956.

(10) —— "The Measurement of Subjective Response." *Qualitative Effects of Drugs.* N.Y., Oxford U. Press, p. 123, 1959.

(11) Benedek, T., "Towards a Biology of a Depressive Constellation." *J. Am. Psychoan. Assn.* 4: 389–427, 1956.

(12) Bergman, H., *Ahad Ha-Am* (Philosophia Judaica Series). Oxford, East and West Library, 1946.

(13) Bowers, M. B., and D. X. Freedman, "Psychedelic Experiences in Acute Psychoses." *Arch. Gen. Psych.* 15: 240–48, 1966.

(14) Bowlby, J., "Processes of Mourning." *Int. J. Psychoan.* 42: 317–40, 1961.

(15) Boyer, L. B., "On Maternal Overstimulation and Ego Defects." *Psychoan. St. Child* 11:236–56, 1956.

(16) Bradley, J. J., "Pain Associated with Depression." *Brit. J. Psych.* 109: 741–45, 1963.

(17) Chein, I., D. L. Gerald, R. S. Lee, and S. Rosenfeld, *The Road to H.* N.Y., Basic Books, 1964.

(18) Chessick, R. D., "The Pharmacogenic Orgasm in Drug Addicts." *Arch. Gen. Psych.* 3: 545–56, 1960.

(19) Chodorkoff, B., "Alcoholism and Ego Function." *Quart. J. St. Alc.* 25: 292–99, 1964.

(20) —— "Body Image Characteristics of the Alcoholics." Mimeographed, Detroit Psychiatric Institute, 1967.

(21) Critchley, M., "Congenital Indifference to Pain." *Arch. Int. Med.* 45: 735–47, 1956.

(22) Dirkman, A. J., "Experimental Meditation." *J. Nerv. & Ment. Dis.* 136: 329–43, 1963.

(23) Dorsey, J. M., Opening Remarks to Second Workshop in *Massive Psychic Trauma,* ed. H. Krystal. N.Y., Int. U. Press, p. 48, 1969.

(24) —— "Vis Medicatrix Naturae." *M.S.M.S.J.* 60: 43–48, 1961.

(25) —— *Illness or Allness.* Detroit, Wayne State U. Press, pp. 44–82, 1965.

(26) ——*Samiska* 9, no. 4, 1955.

(27) ——"Personal Communication" to Seminar on Depression, Detroit General Hosp. and Wayne State U. Dept. of Psychiatry, 1960–61.

(28) Engel, G. L., "Anxiety and Depression—Withdrawal the Primary Affect of Unpleasure." *Int. J. Psychoan.* 43: 89–98, 1962.

(29) Erickson, E. H., "The Problem of Ego Identity," in *Identity and the Life Cycle* (Psych. Issues Monogr. 1). N.Y., Int. U. Press, p. 23, 1959.

(30) Eriksen, C. W., "Perceptual Defense as a Function of Unacceptable Needs." *J. Abn. Soc. Psych.* 46: 283–88, 1951.

(31) Federn, P., *Ego Psychology and the Psychoses.* N.Y., Basic Books, 1945.

(32) Fenichel, O., *The Psychoanalytic Theory of the Neuroses.* N.Y., Norton & Co., 1945.

(33) Fisher, C., "Dreams, Images and Perceptions." *J. Am. Psychoan. Assn.* 4: 5–49, 1956.

(34) Freud, A., "The Role of Bodily Illness in the Mental Life of Children." *Psychoan. St. Child* 7: 69–81, 1952.

(35) Freud, S., *Totem and Taboo.* Standard Edition 13: 60. London, Hogarth Press, 1913.

(36) —— *Mourning and Melancholia.* S.E.14: 245, 1917.

(37) —— *Beyond the Pleasure Principle.* S.E.18: 27, 1920.

(38) ——*Inhibitions, Symptoms and Anxiety.* S.E.20, 1926.
(39) Gardner, R. W., and R. I. Long, "Cognitive Control, Defense and Centration Effect: a Study of Scanning Behavior." *Brit. J. Psych.* 53: 129–40, 1962.
(40) Glover, E., "The Screening Function of Traumatic Memories." *Int. J. Psychoan.* 10: 90–93, 1929.
(41) —— "Common Problems in Psychoanalysis and Anthropology: Drug Ritual and Addiction." *Brit. J. Med. Psychol.* 12: 109–31, 1932.
(42) —— "On the Etiology of Drug Addiction." *Int. J. Psychoan.* 13: 298–328, 1932.
(43) Goldstein, L., "Aspirin vs Anxiety," reported to 1966 Convention of American Societies for Experimental Biology. Quoted in *Modern Medicine,* p. 39, May 23, 1966.
(44) Greenacre, P., *Trauma, Growth and Personality.* N.Y., Norton & Co., pp. 27–83, 1952.
(45) —— "Towards an Understanding of the Physical Nucleus of Some Defense Mechanisms." *Int. J. Psychoan.* 39: 69–76, 1958.
(46) Greenson, R., "On Enthusiasm." *J. Am. Psychoan. Assn.* 10: 3–22, 1962.
(47) Gruber, E. M., *et al.,* "Clinical Bio-essay of Oral Analgesic Activity of Propoxyphrene Acetylic Acid and Codeine Phosphate, and Observations of Placebo Reaction." *Arch. Int. Pharm.* 104: 156–66, 1955.
(48) Hartmann, H., *Essays on Ego Psychology.* N.Y., Int. U. Press, 1964.
(49) ——, E. Kris, and R. M. Lowenstein, "Comments on the Formation of Psychic Structures." *Psychoan. St. Child* 2: 11–39, 1946.
(50) Hill, H. E., C. H. Koznetsky, H. J. Flannery, and A. Wikler, "Studies on Anxiety Associated with Anticipation of Pain." *A.M.A. Arch. Neur. & Psych.* 67: 612–19, 1952.
(51) Jacobson, E., *The Self and the Object World.* N.Y., N.Y.U. Press, 1964.
(52) Kast, E. S., and V. J. Collins, "Lysergic Acid Diethylamine as an Analgesic Agent." *Anesthesia and Analgesia* 43: 285–91, 1964.
(53) Katan, A., "The Role of Displacement in Agoraphobia." *Int. J. Psychoan.* 32: 41–50, 1951.
(54) Keiser, S., "Freud's Concept of Trauma and a Specific Ego Function." *J. Am. Psychoan. Assn.* 15: 781–94, 1967.
(55) Khan, M. M., "The Concept of Cumulative Trauma." *Psychoan. St. Child* 18: 286–307, 1963.

(56) Klein, M., "Notes on Some Schizoid Mechanisms." *Int. J. Psychoan.* 27: 99–110, 1946.

(57) Knapp, P. H., "Sensory Impressions in Dreams." *Psychoan. Quart.* 25: 325–48, 1956.

(58) Kris, E., "The Recovery of Childhood Memories in Psychoanalysis." *Psychoan. St. Child* 11: 54–88, 1956.

(59) Krystal, H., "The Physiological Basis of the Treatment of Delirium Tremens." *Am. J. Psych.* 116: 137–47, 1959.

(60) —— "The Problems of Abstinence by the Patient as a Requisite for the Psychotherapy of Alcoholism." *Quart. J. Studies on Alc.* 23: 105–22, 1962.

(61) —— "The Study of Withdrawal from Narcotics as a State of Stress." *Psych. Quart. Suppl.* 36: 53–65, 1962.

(62) —— "Psychotherapeutic Assistants in the Treatment of Regressed Patients," in *Current Therapies* 4, ed. Jules Masserman. N.Y., Grune and Stratton, 1964.

(63) —— "Withdrawal from Drugs." *Psychosomatics* 7: 299–302, 1966.

(64) —— (ed.), *Massive Psychic Trauma.* N.Y., Int. U. Press, 1968.

(65) —— "Trauma and the Stimulus Barrier," in preparation.

(66) —— and T. A. Petty, "The Psychological Aspects of Normal Convalescence." *Psychosomatics* 2: 1–7, 1961.

(67) Kurland, A. A., S. Unger, and W. N. Pabrinke, "Psychedelic Therapy: Utilizing LSD with Terminal Cancer Patients," Presented to Annual Meeting, Am. Psych. Assn., Detroit, 1967.

(68) Levine, J., and A. Ludwig, "Alterations of Consciousness Produced by Combinations of LSD, Hypnosis and Psychotherapy." *Psychopharmacologia* 7: 123–37, 1965.

(69) Lewin, B., "Mania and Sleep." *Psychoan. Quart.* 18: 419–33, 1949.

(70) Lewin, K., *Phantastica: Die betaubenden und erregenden Genussmittel.* Berlin, Kluge & Co., p. 15, 1929.

(71) Little, M., "On Basic Unity." *Int. J. Psychoan.* 41: 376–84, 1960.

(72) Livingston, W. K., "What is Pain?" *Sc. Amer.* 407: 3–9, 1953.

(73) Loranger, A. U., C. T. Prout, and M. A. White, "The Placebo Effect in Psychiatric Drug Research." *J.A.M.A.* 176: 920–25, 1961.

(74) Ludwig, A., "Altered States of Consciousness." *Arch. Gen. Psych.* 15: 225–34, 1966.

(75) —— and J. Levine, "Alterations in Consciousness Produced by Hypnosis." *J. Nerv. & Ment. Dis.* 140: 146–53, 1965.

(76) Margolis, M., H. Krystal, and S. Siegel, "Psychotherapy with Alcoholic Offenders." *Quart. J. St. Alc.* 25: 85–99, 1964.

(77) May, R., "The Existential Approach in Anxieties." *Am. Textbook of Psych.* N.Y., Basic Books, pp. 1348–61, 1959.

(78) Mayfield, D., and D. Allen, "Alcohol and Affect: Psychopharmacological Study." *Am. J. Psych.* 123: 1346–57, 1967.

(79) Melzack, R., "The Perception of Pain." *Sc. Amer.* 457: 3–12, 1961.

(80) Menninger, K. A., *Man Against Himself.* N.Y., Harcourt, Brace & Co., 1938.

(81) Moore, B. E., "Frigidity in Women." Report of Panel, *J. Am. Psychoan. Assn.* 9: 511–85, 1961.

(82) Moore, R. A., "Reaction-Formation as a Countertransference Phenomenon in the Treatment of Alcoholics." *Quart. J. Studies on Alc.* 22: 481–86, 1961.

(83) Murphy, W. F., "Character, Trauma and Sensory Perception." *Int. J. Psychoan.* 39: 535–69, 1958.

(84) ―― "Trauma and Loss." *J. Am. Psychoan. Assn.* 9: 519–32, 1961.

(85) McCleary, J. E., and H. M. Lazarus, in J. Bucuner and O. Kurch, *Perception and Personality.* Durham, Duke U. Press, 1949.

(86) McGinnies, E., "Emotionality and Perceptual Defense." *Psychol. Rev.* 56: 244–51, 1949.

(87) Nacht, S., and S. Viderman, "Pre-Object Universe in the Psychoanalytic Situation." *Int. J. Psychoan.* 41: 385–88, 1960.

(88) Niederland, W. G., "The Problem of the Survivor." *J. Hillside Hosp.* 10: 233–96, 1961.

(89) Novey, S., "The Meaning of the Concept of Mental Representation of Objects." *Psychoan. Quart.* 27: 58–80, 1958.

(90) Nunberg, H., *Principles of Psychoanalysis.* N.Y., Int. U. Press, p. 51, 1955.

(91) Olds, J., "Pleasure Centers in the Brain." *Sc. Amer.* 30: 1–8, 1956.

(92) Ostow, M., "Psychic Function of Temporal Lobes as Inferred from Seizure Phenomena." *Arch. Neur. & Psych.* 77: 79–85, 1957.

(93) ―― *Drugs in Psychoanalysis and Psychotherapy.* N.Y., Basic Books, 1962.

(94) Petrie, A., *Individuality in Pain and Suffering.* Chicago, U. of Chicago Press, 1967.

(95) Rado, S., "The Psychoanalysis of Pharmacothymia." *Psych. Quart.* 2: 2–23, 1935.

(96) Ramzy, I., and R. S. Wallerstein, "Pain, Fear and Anxiety: a Study in their Interrelationship." *Psychoan. St. Child* 13: 147–89, 1958.

(97) Rangell, L., "The Metapsychology of Trauma," in S. Furst's *Psychic Trauma*. N.Y., Basic Books, pp. 51–85, 1967.

(98) Rapaport, D., *Emotions and Memory*. N.Y., Int. U. Press, p. 22, 1950.

(99) —— "Consciousness: A Psychopathological and Psychodynamic View," in *Problems of Consciousness*. N.Y., J. Macy Found., p. 20, 1957.

(100) Raskin, H. A., "Rehabilitation of the Narcotic Addict." *J.A.M.A.* 189: 956–58, 1964.

(101) ——, T. A. Petty, and M. Warren, "A Suggested Approach to the Problem of Narcotic Addiction." *Am. J. Psych.* 113: 1089–94, 1957.

(102) Rees, J. R., *The Shaping of Psychiatry by War*. N.Y., Norton & Co., 1945.

(103) Savitt, R. A., "Psychoanalytic Studies on Addiction: Ego Structure in Narcotic Addicts." *Psychoan. Quart.* 32: 43–57, 1963.

(104) Schecheheye, C. F., *Symbolic Realization*. N.Y., Int. U. Press, 1951.

(105) Schur, M., "Comments on the Metapsychology of Somatization." *Psychoan. St. Child* 10: 119–64, 1955.

(106) Selzer, M. L., "Hostility as a Barrier to Therapy in Alcoholism." *Psych. Quart.* 31: 301–05, 1957.

(107) Shor, R. E., "The Frequency of Naturally Occurring 'Hypnoid-like' Experiences in the Normal College Population." *Int. J. Clin. & Exp. Hypn.* 8: 151–63, 1960.

(108) Silverman, J. A., "A Paradigm for the Study of Altered States of Consciousness." *Brit. J. Psych.* 114: 1201–18, 1968.

(109) Solnit, A., and M. Kris, "Trauma and Infantile Experiences: a Longitudinal Perspective," in S. Furst's *Psychic Trauma*. N.Y., Basic Books, pp. 175–221, 1967.

(110) Sterba, R., *Introduction to the Psychoanalytic Theory of the Libido*. N.Y., Nervous and Mental Disorders Monogr., 1947.

(111) Stern, M. M., "Anxiety, Trauma and Shock." *Psychoan. Quart.* 20: 179–203, 1951.

(112) —— "Fear of Death and Neurosis." *J. Am. Psychoan. Assn.* 16: 3–31, 1968.

(113) —— "Fear of Death and Trauma." *Int. J. Psychoan.* 49: 458–61, 1968.

(114) Szasz, T., *Pain and Pleasure*. London, Tavistock, p. 77, 1957.

(115) —— "The Counterphobic Mechanism in Addiction." *J. Am. Psychoan. Assn.* 6: 309–25, 1958.

(116) Weiss, J., "Intensity as a Character Trait." *Psychoan. Quart.* 28: 64–72, 1959.

(117) Wetmore, R. J., "The Role of Grief in Psychoanalysis." *Int. J. Psychoan.* 44: 97–104, 1963.

(118) Winnicott, D. W., "Mind and its Relation to Psyche-Soma" (1949). *Collected Papers.* N.Y., Basic Books, 1958.

(119) Wolf, H. G., J. P. Hardy, and H. Goodell, "Studies in Pain." *J. Clin. Invest.* 19: 659–88, 1940.

(120) Wolf, S., and R. H. Pinsky, "Effect of Placebo Administration and Occurrence of Toxic Reaction." *J.A.M.A.* 135: 339–41, 1942.

(121) World Health Organization Expert Committee on Addiction-Producing Drugs. Seventh Report, W. H. O. Technical Report Service 116: 9, 1957.

addendum

(122) Eddy, N., *et al.*, "Drug Dependence: Its Significance and Characteristics." *Psychopharmacology Bull.* 3: 1–12, July 1966.

index

Acute psychosis, 84
Addict. *See* Drug dependent
"Addiction," 9. *See also* Drug dependence
Adolescence, 107
Affects, 32; consciousness of, 23; desomatized, 16, 24; developmental history of, 20–22; differentiation of, 38; as drive derivatives, 99; drugs and generation of, 73; genetic view of, 15 *ff.*; primitivization of, 20; regression and, 104 (*see also* De-differentiation; Deverbalization; Resomatization); as signal, 30–31; verbalization of, 16, 87. *See also* Drug dependent; Unpleasant; Ur-affects
Affect tolerance, 32–33
Aggression: and anxiety, 15–16; in counter-transference, 103; dealing with, 109–10; dread of own, 51, 104–5; in infancy, 19, 51, 67–68; mastery of, 101; repressed, 52, 61–63, 65; toward mother or self, 52; toward object-representation, 55
Aggressive energy, 57–58
Agnosia, congenital pain, 16–17
Ahad Ha-Am, 54
Alcohol: desire for 60, 63; effects of, 80, 85–86; and psychotherapy, 98
Alcoholic hallucinosis, 78, 102

Alcoholics, 41, 77, 85, 91, 102; changes in body-image of, 37; Clyde-Mood scale, 74–75; denial in, 67; and love objects, 48; and perception, 34
Allen, D., 74, 85
"Altered states of consciousness," 75–78, 82
Ambivalence: toward drug, 103; toward early love objects, 67; libido and aggression, 51; toward lost love object (*see* Loss; Mourning); toward love object, 47; toward object-representation (-relation), 48, 49, 66; toward physician, 46
Amnesia, functional, 79
Amphetamines, 86, 88; and anxiety-agitation response, 22; and other stimulants, 34
Analgesia, 95
Analgesic action of drugs, 39
Analgesics, 45–46
Anesthesia, 85–86, 92, 95
Annihilation: dread of, 56; threat of, 67
Antabuse, 59; used in therapy, 98, 102, 103
Anxiety: as affect of pain, 24; "agitation" in, 22; and alcohol, 85; characterizes traumatized individual, 17; close relationship to pain, 15–16, 19, 29; in concentration camp survivors, 17;

de-differentiated from depression, 22; and depersonalization, 27–28; homosexual panic, 98–99; in infant, 20–21; infantile versus adult form of, 24 (*see also* Desomatization; Differentiation; Verbalization); lack of stimuli causes, 40; libidinization of, 39; and masculine functions, 92; medical, 81; mobilized, 16; neurotic, 88; in normal people, 17; and object-representation, 16; and pain, 24–25; related to drug dependence, 15–16; as signal, 24, 31, 91 n; in soldiers, 18; and wakefulness, alertness, 86; warded off, 81. *See also* Pain

Anxiety, relief of: aspirin, 19; morphine and narcotic analgesics, 18; placebo, 46. *See also* Drugs, uses

Anxiety-depression, 33, 35, 86

Arlow, J., 65

Aspirin and anxiety, 19

Bak, R. C., 55

Barbiturates, uses of, 38–39

Beecher, H. K., 45–46

Benedek, T., 25

Body function, modification of, 93–95, 96

Body-image, 76, 78, 80, 92–95

"Borderline" patients, 100. *See also* Schizophrenics

Boredom, 73, 77, 91

Bowers, M. B., 84

Bowlby, J., 40

Boyer, L. B., 36

Brenner, R., 65

Cannabis, 88, 111

Cathexes, shift of, 84–85

"Cathexis of mental energy," 49

Central nervous system, 41–42

"Centration effect," 82

Chein, I., 12, 33, 48

Chessick, R. D., 26

Chodorkoff, B., 37

Clyde-Mood scale, 74

CNS, 41–42

Codeine, 46

Cognition, 86; modification of, 76 *ff.*; pre-conscious mode of, 84–85; primary process, 81; suppression of critical, 95. *See also* Perception

"Congenital analgesic indifference," 17

Consciousness, 75–79, 82, 84; blocked, 87; disorientation of, 79; modification of, 13, 75 *ff. See also* Body-image; Ego; Perception; Self-awareness

Constancy principle, 40, 42

Conversion of drug user, 106

Counter-cathectic energy, 28

Counter-cathexis, 65, 91; of aggressive impulses, 68

"Counter-irritation," 28

Counter-transference, 101, 103

"Crying in one's beer," 76, 89, 91

Cultural patterns for dealing with pain and unpleasant affects, 25–26

De-differentiation: of affects, 30; as regression in regard to affects, 20; of underlying fantasies, 104

Demerol, 92

Deneutralization (erotization) of affects, 36

Depersonalization, 76; as defense against anxiety or pain, 27–28; as hysterical conversion symptom, 28

Depressed patients, 74, 84

Depression, 52, 67, 77; and alcohol, 85; chronic, 89, 90;

Depression (*con't.*)
  differentiated and de-differentiated from anxiety, 21–22; manic defense against, 86; in mourning, 52, 55; and pain, 26; warded off, 81
Desomatization: of affect, 16, 24; response, 23
Destructive fantasies, 27
Deutsch, H., 43
Deverbalization, 20
Differentiation of affects, 38. *See also* Desomatization; Verbalization
Dirkman, A. J., 82
Discharge of: drives, 40, 43; impulses, 40; pleasure, 44; tension, 42
Disorganization, 40–41
Disorientation, 96; and alcoholics, 85; of consciousness, 79
Dissociation, 79–80, 96
Distress patterns, 20–21, 38. *See also* De-differentiation
Dorsey, J. M., 29, 53, 64, 71, 73
Drive discharge, 40, 43
Drug dependence: adaptive and functional, 12; and adolescents, 12; change in terminology, 10; counterphobic attitudes in, 39; defined, 10; ego syntonic, 12; etiology, 10–11; as extreme form of transference, 71; and libidinization of anxiety, 39; as medical syndrome and symptom complex, 11; as mental or emotional disorder, 11; reaction to withdrawal symptoms, 37; related to anxiety, 15–16; specific relief sought by, 44; and trauma, 30–31 (see also Traumatization); when a major problem, 108
Drug dependent: ability for self-

distraction impaired in, 28; adolescents, 12; as chronic suicide, 109; desires fusion with object, 48, 57, 58; disturbed relationship to love object, 47–48 (*see also* Object-representation); dreads primary pleasure affects, 33; intolerant of anxiety, 30; needs immediate gratification, 30; not aware of own affects, 26; and physiological regression, 23; regression in regard to affects, 20; resistance to trauma defective in, 31 (*see also* Stimulus barrier); seeks relief of painful states, 15; schizoid personality type, 41
Drugs: amphetamine-like, 38; and central nervous system, 41; depressant, 9; effects of, 82, 84–85; hallucinogenic, 9; psychotropic, 37; and regression, 40; short- versus long-acting, 58; stimulant, 9; sympatho-mimetic, 18; tolerance of, 9, 10. *See also specific drugs*
Drugs, uses of, 111–12: to adjust to loss of love object, 49 (*see also* Loss); anhedonic, 108; to avoid boredom and unpleasant affects, 73, 95–96, 108 (*see also* Tolerance; to avoid impending psychic trauma, 31; for dissociation, 79–80; to modify consciousness, 75 *ff.* (*see also* Disorientation; Dissociation; Modification); as mother-substitute, 103; as object-substitute, 47–48; to relieve tension, 48; to relieve Ur-affects, 34; as self-help, 11; to suppress reflective self-awareness, 88; as transference object, 45; as transubstantiation, 48
Dysphoric affect, 86; states, 35–36

Economic principle, 43
Ecstatic states, 75, 95; religious, 88–89
Eddy, N., 10, 119
Ego, 48, 52, 65, 91, 91 n, 92, 97; and affects, 13; and consciousness, 78; development of, 24; function of, 49; impoverished, 70; modified, 89, 92; and object-representation, 13; overwhelmed, 32; and self-representation, 13; threatened by aggressive impulses, 51. *See also* Consciousness; Modification; Object-, Self-representation
Ego dysfunction, 13
Ego functions, 32, 38, 78, 80, 84, 102, 104; dependent on love object, 40; disturbance of, 98; and drug dependence, 11–12, 13, 15; handling unpleasant affects, 29; imperfect development of, 108; impaired, 35, 111; infant's lack of, 20; involved in mastery and tolerance of pain, 28; necessity of objects for, 40; and therapy, 100
Ego ideal, 89, 92; identity, 50; psychology, 12
Emotional expressiveness, 76
Engel, G. L., 22
Erickson, E. H., 50
Erotization of affects, 36
Excitation pattern, 30
Externalization of object-representation, 65, 68; case illustrations, 58–64

"False insight," 84
Fantasy fusion, 68
Fechner, G. T., 40
Federn, P., 49
Fenichel, O., 50, 52, 106
Fisher, C., 81

Food as symbol, 59. *See also* Hunger
Freedman, D. X., 84
Freud, A. 19, 24–25
Freud, S., 23, 29, 31, 40, 43, 52, 54, 55, 91
Fusion, oceanic, 69, 76, 80
Fusion of self- and object-representations, 65–66, 88; in alcoholics, 57; case illustrations, 58–64; in drug dependents, 48, 57–58; in LSD users, 58; in schizophrenics, 56–57. *See also* Fantasy; Introjection; Nirvana

Gerard, D. L., 12
Ginsberg, Allen, 69–70
Glover, E., 40
Goldstein, L., 18–19
Greenacre, P., 37
Greenson, R., 47
Group therapy, 97
Guilt, infant's sense of, 19

Hallucinations, auditory, 92
Hallucinatory experiences, 80, 85; pre-verbal, 94
Hallucinogenic drugs, 9
"Hangover," 47–48
Hartmann, H., 50
Heroin user, 86, 92
Hunger as symbol, 63, 87, 105. *See also* Food
Hypercathexis, 37, 57; of perceptual system, 93–94
Hypersuggestibility, 78
Hypnosis, 80
"Hypnotical phenomena," 83
Hypnotic method, 95; states, 75
Hypnotics, use of, 105
Hypocathexis, 86
Hypomanic state, 63

Iatrogenic addicts, 26

Impulses, mastery of, 101
Incestuous tie, 94, 107. *See also* Love object; Mother; Object-representation
Incorporative yearnings. *See* Fusion; Introjection; Nirvana
Indifference, 17, 86
Individuation, process of, 48
Infancy: aggression in, 19, 67–68; anxiety in, 20–21, 24; discovery of love object, 20–21; distress patterns of, 20–21; lack of ego functions in, 20; orgasm in, 42; oral stage of, 87; and pain, 19–20; reaction to loss in, 23; rejection in, 52; sense of guilt in, 19; stimulus barrier in, 19; trauma in, 17, 19, 33; and Ur-affects, 22, 31. *See also* Mother
Infantile satiation-fusion, 58
Instinct gratification, 99–100
Introjection of object-representation, 51–52, 55, 58, 70, 87

Jacobson, E., 50, 51

Katan, A., 107
Keiser, S., 35
Khan, M. M., 19, 37–38
Khat, 88
Klein, M., 21, 51
Knapp, P. H., 93
Korsakoff, F. S., 77
Kris, E., 36 n. 50
Krystal, H., 10, 20, 22, 27, 37, 57, 97, 98, 99, 101, 102, 108
Kurland, A. A., 88

Lee, R. S., 12
Levine, J., 80
Lewin, B., 87, 106
Libidinal energy, 57
Libidinization of anxiety, 39

Libido, 51
Little, M., 56
Livingston, W. K., 27
Loss of love object, 55, 107, 110; inability of alcoholics and drug users to adjust to, 48; and object-representation, 52–55; threat of, 20–21, 67. *See also* Mourning
Love object, 106–07; ambivalence toward, 47; disappointment with, 70; discovery of, in infancy, 20–21; disturbed relationship of drug dependent with, 47–48; dysfunction of maternal, 36–38; early, 67; and ego functions, 40; incestuous, 94; mother as, 19–21; placebo as substitute for, 47; threat of loss of, 20–21, 67. *See also* Object-representation
Lowenstein, R., 50
LSD (lysergic acid diethylamide), 58, 69; "effects," 80; effects of, 82–83, 93
Ludwig, A., 75–78, 80

McGinnies, E., 81
Manic defenses, 86
Maternal function, 36–38
Mayfield, D., 74, 85
"Medically addicted" individuals, 26
Melzack, R., 16
Memory, 90–91; as stimulus, 32. *See also* Trauma
Menninger, K., 109
Modification: of body function, 93–95, 96; of body-image, 76, 80, 92–95; of consciousness, 13, 75–78, 82; of interpretation of event, 88–89; of orientation, 79–85; of pain experience, 27 (*see also* Tolerance); of perception, 34, 76, 80–83; of self-awareness

and superego function, 88–93; of wakefulness, 85–87

Morphine, 18, 45. *See also* Opiates

Mother, 36–38, 105; childhood aggression toward, 63; death of, 66–67; as love object, 19–21, 71; repressed, 68; role in child's experiencing pain, 25; and self-identity, 68. *See also* Infancy; Loss; Love

Mourning, 40; analogy to, 107; effect on object-representation, 52–55; effect on self-representation, 53–55; pain in, 55; psychic pain in, 28; when impossible, 66–67. *See also* Loss

Murphy, W. F., 34, 93

Nacht, S., 56

Narcissism, 93; and object-representation, 48, 51, 70; secondary, 49–50

Narcotic analgesics, 18

Narcotics, 9; dependence on, 97–98; and pain, 26

Neurotics, 94, 100

Nirvana, fusion with, 33, 48, 69

Norepinephrine release, 38, 88

Novey, S., 49

"Object-addiction," 106

Object-representation (-relation), 20, 48 *ff.*, 104; and anxiety, 16; case illustrations, 58–64; created by patient, 106; development of, 50–52; and ego, 13; introjection of, 51, 52, 55, 58, 70, 87; maintaining, outside self, 63; and mourning, 52–55 (*see also* Loss); narcissistic nature of, 48, 51, 70; and self-representation, 50–52. *See also* Fusion; Self-

Object-substitute, 58, 64, 71; drug

as, 105, 111; loss of, 103

Oblivion, 33

Olds, J., 41

Opiates, 12; as analgesics, 45; and Nirvana, 33

Oral fantasies, 103; frustration, 52; gratification, 21; stage of infancy, 87

Orgasm, 41–43

Osler, W., 46

Ostow, M., 26

Pain: and anxiety, 15–17, 19, 24–25, 29; in children, 19–20, 24–25; conscious and complex process, 27; and "counter-irritation," 28; depersonalization as defense, 27–28; and depression, 26; hyperreactivity and hyporeactivity to, 17; and morphine, 18; in mourning, 55; and narcotic analgesics, 18; nature of, 23–24; perception of, 26 *ff.*; as perceptive process, 24–25; physical, 55, 86; as return of traumatic situation, 17; secondary process in experiencing, 27; threshold, 18, 32. *See also* Tolerance; Trauma

Paranoid, 78

Perception: identified with object, 94; modified by drugs, 34, 76, 80–83; of pain, 26 *ff.*; pleasurable, 87; and "psychedelic" drugs, 94; self-, impaired by drugs, 74 (*see also* Ego; Self-); sensory, 80–81, 93

Petrie, A., 80

Petty, T. A., 27, 30

Pharmacogenic orgasm, 41–42

"Pharmacothymic crisis," 102

Physical pain, 55, 86

Physiological regression, 23

Placebo, 45–47, 80

Pleasure, 40

Pleasure principle, 78; modified, 42–44

Pre-object state, 50

Proprioception, 21

"Psychedelic" drugs, 85, 95; "experiences," 84, 94. *See also* LSD

Psychic trauma and affects, 31–32

Psychoanalysis, 26, 53

Psychosis, acute, 84

Psychotherapy, 80, 97 *ff.*; causes of need for, 110–12; evaluating drug user for, 110; with narcotics and alcohol dependents, 26; types of, 107–8

Psychotic "anxiety," 21; "insight," 76; (toxic) states, 75–76

Psychotics, 100

Psychotropic drugs, 37

Rado, S., 22, 41, 102

Rapaport, D., 77, 78

Raskin, H. A., 30, 48

Reality "perception," 49; testing, 78

Rejection in childhood, 52, 59–60

Rejuvenation, feeling of, 77

Relief principle, 43

Religious ecstasy, 88–89

Repression, 53, 64 *ff.*, 91 n; of aggression, 52, 61–63, 65; of impulses, "breakthrough," 84; of selfness, 65

Resomatization, 20. *See also* De-differentiation

Reunion, desire for, 69–70

Rosenfeld, E., 12

Savitt, R. A., 48

Schizoid personality types, 40–41

Schizophrenics, 51, 55–57; versus drug users, 94–95

Schur, M., 23

Secondary process in experiencing pain, 27

Self-awareness: painful, 95; reflective, 87. *See also* Ego

Self-identity: awakening to ("tertiary process"), 53–54; and mother, 68

Selfness, repression of, 65

Self-perception and drugs, 74

Self-representation, 20, 48 *ff.*; development of, 50; effect of mourning on, 53–55; and ego, 13; impoverishment of, 65; modification of, 94; and object-representation, 50–52. *See also* Ego; Fusion; Object-

Self-stimulation, 41–42

Sensory perception, 80–81, 93

Sherrington, C., 27

Shor, R. E., 83–84

Silverman, J. A., 80–81, 82, 83

Solipsim, 54

Somnolence, 85–87

Sterba, R., 49

Stimulants, 9

Stimuli: lack of, 40; and maternal function, 36–38; memories as, 32; not consciously recognized, 81; perception of, 32; reaction to, 82–83; relief from unpleasant, 42–43

Stimulus barrier, 29, 31 *ff.*; and drugs, 33 *ff.*; heightened, 83; infant's, 19; and traumatization syndrome, 32 (*see also* Trauma)

Stimulus threshold and tolerance, 32

Strain-trauma, 36

Studies of drug effects, 74–75

"Subception," 81

Suicide, 86, 103; and addiction 109; attempts, 68

Superego: blocking of, 95; ex-

ternalization of, 67, 97; function suspended, 91–92
Sympatho-mimetic drugs, 18
Szasz, T., 29, 39

Tachistoscopic studies, 81
Tension: accumulation and discharge of, 42–44; awareness of, 95; and drugs, 48; intersystemic, 76; tolerance of, 44; wish for relief of, 87
"Tertiary process," 53–54
Therapist, 67, 98 *ff.*; "chief," 57; schizophrenics and, 56–57
Thresholds: of pain, 18, 32; of pleasure and unpleasure, 40; of trauma resistance, 17
"Thrills," 39, 88
Tolerance of pain (unpleasant affects), 28, 32, 38, 47, 88, 99, 102, 108, 109; development of, in children, 24–25; ego functions and, 28; drugs and reduction of, 28
Toxic (psychotic) states, 75–76
Tranquilizers, uses of, 91
Transference, 61, 66, 98, 103; in alcoholics and drug dependents, 57; counter-, 101, 103; and drug dependence, 71; object, drug as, 45; in psychotherapy, 57–58; in schizophrenics, 56–57; use of, 106
Transubstantiation of object, 70, 106; drug as, 48; introjection of, 69. *See also* Object-substitute
Trauma: "automatic anxiety" in, 21; and concentration camp survivors, 17; cumulative, 37; and drug dependence, 30–31; economic concept, 29; fear of return of, 36, 105, 110; in infancy and prenatal period, 17, 19; infant's fear of after affects

of, 33; phenomenon of, 29–30; states, 82; strain-, 36; syndrome, 21; threat of, 24; threshold of resistance of, 17
Traumatic process, 30; screen, 17, 32; situation, 17, 33; essence of, 29
Traumatization, 43, 91, 111; massive psychic, 17; syndrome, 32
Traumatized individual: drug user as, 110; hyperreactive to pain, 17

Union. *See* Fusion; Nirvana
Unpleasant affect (pain), relief of, 75–76, 85, 95–96. *See also* Affects; Pain; Tolerance
Unpleasure, 40; blocked, 87; primary affect of, 22; relief of, 43; threshold of, 40; Ur-affects of, 70. *See also* Pain
Ur-affects: of anxiety-depression, 33; and infants, 22, 31; "numbing" and blocking of, 34; precursor of anxiety and depression, 20; relief of, 34, 38 *ff.*; resomatized, 24; in therapy, 100; of unpleasure, 70

Verbalization of affect, 16, 87; aspect of ego development, 24. *See also* Differentiation
Viderman, S., 56

Wakefulness, 85–87, 95
Warren, M., 30
Wetmore, R. J., 53
Winnicott, D. W., 37
Wish-fulfillment, 44, 76–77, 92; fantasy, 88
Withdrawal, 57, 108; states, 20, 101; symptoms, 37; syndrome, 9, 10
World Health Organization, 9

Henry Krystal and Herbert A. Raskin are adjunct associate professors of psychiatry, Wayne State University, and hold other professional academic appointments. In addition, they are general practicing psychoanalysts. Dr. Krystal, a native of Gleiwitz, Poland, earned his M.D. from Wayne State University Medical School in 1953, and edited *Massive Psychic Trauma,* published in 1969.

Dr. Raskin, a native of Detroit, also received his M.D. from Wayne State University (1949). Both doctors have published widely in professional journals.

Charles H. Elam edited the manuscript. The book was designed by Mary Jowski. The text type used is Mergenthaler's Times Roman, designed by Stanley Morison in 1929. The display type face is Helvetica.

The book is printed on Warren's Olde Style Antique paper. The book is bound in Columbia Mills' Bayside Vellum cloth over binder's boards. Manufactured in the United States of America.